307.140973
Ar2i

131395

DATE DUE			

Implementing
change in communities
A COLLABORATIVE PROCESS

Implementing change in communities

A COLLABORATIVE PROCESS

SARAH ELLEN ARCHER, R.N., Dr.PH.

Professor and Coordinator,
Community Health Nursing, School of Nursing,
University of California, San Francisco, California

CAROLE D. KELLY, R.N., M.S.

Visiting Lecturer, Community Health Nursing,
School of Nursing, University of California,
San Francisco, California

President, Nursing Dynamics Corporation,
Mill Valley, California

SALLY ANN BISCH, R.N., M.S. (Hyg)

Candidate, Doctor of Nursing Science,
International and Cross-cultural Nursing,
School of Nursing, University of California,
San Francisco, California

Illustrated

CARL A. RUDISILL LIBRARY
LENOIR RHYNE COLLEGE

The C. V. Mosby Company

ST. LOUIS   TORONTO   1984

MOSBY

A TRADITION OF PUBLISHING EXCELLENCE

Editor: Alison Miller
Assistant editor: Susan Epstein
Manuscript editor: Diane Ackermann
Design: Jeanne Bush
Production: Jeanne Gulledge, Mary Stueck

Copyright © 1984 by The C.V. Mosby Company

All rights reserved. No part of this publication may be reproduced,
stored in a retrieval system, or transmitted, in any form or by any
means, electronic, mechanical, photocopying, recording, or otherwise,
without prior written permission from the publisher.

Printed in the United States of America

The C.V. Mosby Company
11830 Westline Industrial Drive, St. Louis, Missouri 63146

Library of Congress Cataloging in Publication Data

Archer, Sarah Ellen.
  Implementing change in communities.

  Bibliography: p.
  Includes index.
  1. Community development—United States.
2. Community organization—United States. 3. Social
indicators—United States.   I. Kelly, Carole D.
II. Bisch, Sally Ann.   III. Title. [DNLM: 1. Community
health services—Organization and administration.
2. Social planning. 3. Social change. 4. Group
processes. 5. Health services for the aged—Organization and administration. WA 546.1 A 672i]
HN90.C6A76   1984   307'.14'0973   83-17354
ISBN 0-8016-0300-5

AC/VH/VH 9 8 7 6 5 4 3 2 1   01/D/052

FOREWORD

In this era of competition models, is it impractical and idealistic to write a book accurately titled *Implementing Change in Communities: A Collaborative Process?* Or is it not only hopeful, but sensible—a much-needed guide for practitioners in the fields of health and human services? I vote for the latter; not simply because of my own philosophical bent, but because here I have read something that is highly pragmatic, based on a strong theoretical framework—a way to go forward. The authors have done what they write about, and the reader can benefit from the positive experiences as well as the freely-admitted errors. They are educators and practitioners in the field, and they have combined these roles in a way that can be a model for others.

Although all are nurses, their orientation is public health in the broad sense, and the content of this book is eminently useful to other disciplines. Each chapter has a theoretical framework that is brought alive by examples that clearly illustrate the concepts—all in readable prose. The final chapters of real case studies with accompanying sections that present some of the specific tools are particularly useful. Another interesting component is the well-researched historical background of some topics such as social indicators.

The writers' own philosophy about dealing with the community and other disciplines is self-evident from the title but nicely illustrated in a number of ways. For instance, one seldom hears much about the ethics of consultation and evaluation as is discussed in those chapters. In addition, at a time when many seem to see other disciplines and the opposite sex as enemies to be defeated, it is refreshing to have demonstrated that collaboration and reasonable flexibility can take one further in achieving one's goal (and incidentally, that of the community that is being served).

As a teacher, I expect to find that this book meets many of the educational needs of my varied students in public health. As someone sitting on boards and committees of community agencies, I look forward to sharing it with my co-members. For whether it is used as a textbook or a field reference, this book can assist us in putting into a reality framework the belief that "planned change is legitimate and possible and can help communities and aggregates move toward a desired future."

Lucie S. Kelly, R.N., Ph.D., F.A.A.N.,

Professor of Public Health and Nursing,
School of Public Health and School of Nursing,
Columbia University

PREFACE

This book is designed to provide students and practitioners in health and human service disciplines with a guide for collaborative processes for implementing community change. We include nurses, ministers, community mental health workers, directors, board members of community agencies, health planners, attorneys, social workers, and others who practice in community settings, both domestic and international. Activists, grant writers, researchers, and educators will also find it helpful. The book can be used as a text for students in both undergraduate and graduate courses as well as a field reference for practitioners in a variety of community settings.

The authors have experience in community health nursing, community mental health, education, research, and consultation at local, state, national, and international levels. The perspectives we bring to this book are shaped by these backgrounds. We are philosophically committed to a collaborative consultation model that involves community and aggregate members throughout the process. We believe that planned change is legitimate and possible and can help communities and aggregates move toward a desired future. Our experience has shown us that evaluation components must be built into all phases of planned change. We have often found ourselves either drowning in information and data or unable to find anything we could use.

We have written a textbook and field guide addressing these and other issues that we and others can use to work more effectively with communities and aggregates. Collaboration is the umbrella concept that overrides and pervades all others. The theoretical underpinnings of the book are from systems theory, holism, and social indicators research. Community organization, consultation, planning, change, and evaluation are the processes we describe to facilitate collaboratively implemented change. These relationships are illustrated in Fig. A.

Our focus throughout is on community systems and subsystems, or aggregates, rather than on one-to-one client services. Communities have many definitions. The communities to which we make reference here are primarily geopolitical units such as cities, counties, or states. All people, agencies, organizations, institutions, and other subsystems within these geopolitical jurisdictions are part of "the community." Thus communities are often large pluralistic entities with complex interrelationships and even more complex needs and wants. Aggregates, in our context, are subsystems of communities; they are generally smaller and may be more loosely bound together

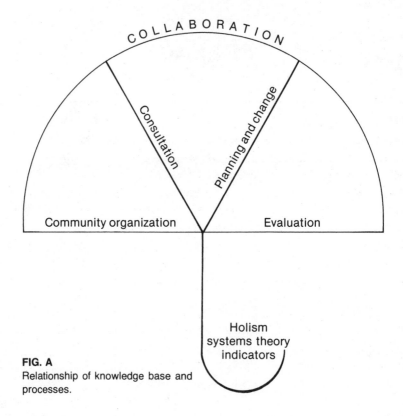

FIG. A
Relationship of knowledge base and
processes.

than are communities. For example, the elderly aggregate, on which our case studies focus, is a relatively loosely associated aggregate.

OBJECTIVES

Again, the overriding goal for this book is to help people in health and human services to work more effectively in collaborative planning for community change. Our more specific objectives are:

1. To bring together an overview of many of the theories and processes that are useful in working with communities and aggregates
2. To assist faculty who teach community health nursing, community medicine, community assessment, planning, or related courses at both undergraduate and graduate levels to help their students to focus on communities and aggregates rather than on individuals
3. To provide people working in domestic and international communities with a practical guidebook that can be used as a reference
4. To stimulate community workers to look beyond direct one-to-one client services to larger community systems where they can help to effect change

OVERVIEW OF THE BOOK

We have organized the book with the following conceptual model in mind:

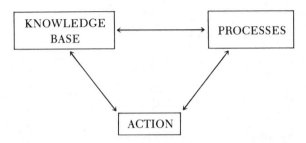

The conceptual model is based on systems theory. As such, all three of its parts are interrelated and interdependent; each provides the other with feedback. Each of the three subsystems is strengthened by the other two, and the total output from all three far exceeds the mere sum of the parts. Systems theory is also a holistic theory, since its focus is on total aggregates, organizations, and communities.

Our discussions of systems, holism, and social and health indicators provide the background for the processes of planning, community organization, consultation, and evaluation that we need in collaborative work for community change (see Fig. 1, p. 16). We conclude with detailed descriptions of two community planning and evaluation examples. These case studies coupled with the numerous examples throughout the rest of the book are its action component.

Concepts from general systems theory and holism are the major content of Chapter 1, the keystone of our conceptual framework. Our model for collaboration is based on Sally Bisch's research. It consists of two systems that we usually associate with planned change: the consultant/planner/evaluator system and the community/aggregate/target system. The collaborative processes we discuss and describe for bringing about planned changes occur within a third system, which is formed by the interrelationships of the other two systems (see Fig. 1, p. 16). This new system is the collaborative intersystem, which has a character and life of its own.

Chapter 2 is devoted to planning and change process. Planning is defined as a collaborative, orderly, and cyclic process used to attain a mutually agreed-on desired future. The outcomes of the planning process involve change, and these changes and their consequences must be evaluated. Decision trees and program evaluation review technique (PERT) networks are offered as examples of planning tools. Change, a component of almost all planning outcomes, is presented from these perspectives. First-order change, that is, change within existing systems and their rules, and second-order change, which is change in the system, call for the development of new rules. Finally, change is dealt with as unfinished business that must be kept flexible rather than being refrozen.

Chapter 3 contains a discussion of selected theories of community organization.

The principles of community organization are made clearer by an example of a grass-roots–organizing project that Carole Kelly participated in when a local nursing home was closed, which created a crisis in a community that already had too few nursing home beds.

We introduce consultation in Chapter 4 with a review of the literature, including some of the salient research that has been done. We discuss a six-step consultation process. Consultation examples in domestic and international settings are given. We stress throughout that consultation is a collaborative process between consultant and consultee and that both are changed through their interaction. We close with some ethical considerations and some thoughts on marketing our consultation skills.

In Chapter 5 evaluation of collaborative efforts at community change has five components: needs assessment, evaluation of alternative courses of action, formative evaluation, summative evaluation, and evaluation of the consequent impacts on the community. Research designs and methods as well as issues of protection of human subjects and informed consent are represented in the context of their use in evaluating community change efforts.

Chapter 6 focuses on social indicators and the social indicator movement. Definitions and characteristics of social indicators and social indices are given. Social indicators are discussed from a number of perspectives including quality of data, relation to other variables, breadth of comparability, and usefulness. The Physical Quality of Life Index is used as an example.

The two case studies in Chapters 7 and 8 are extensive examples of our work in specific communities with elderly aggregates. We discuss the processes used and what we learned. We share many of our mistakes so that our readers will be able to avoid at least some of them.

The final bibliography is mainly for those who want to do more reading on the theories and strategies presented.

All in all, the book is a mix of the practical and the theoretical, experiences and concepts. The two are inextricable; neither alone is adequate. All three of us share a primary commitment to working collaboratively with people to help bring about change. Carole Kelly and Sarah Archer are practical and pragmatic as the case studies in Chapters 7 and 8 illustrate. Sally Bisch is an excellent conceptualizer. To her we owe the collaborative system model that is the unifying theme for the book.

The opinions and ideas expressed here are ours. We take full responsibility for them. Our blend of theory and practice, knowledge and experience, is the product of our shared backgrounds. Our collaboration has greatly enriched and changed us all, as collaboration always does. We hope what we have learned and now pass on to you is of some use.

Sarah Ellen Archer
Carole D. Kelly
Sally Ann Bisch

ACKNOWLEDGMENTS

No one can ever acknowledge all of the people and organizations that contribute to a work like this. We owe inestimable debts to literally thousands of people in the communities and aggregates in the United States and in other countries with whom we have been privileged to work and from whom we have learned so much. All of us have had faculty whose courses and personal examples have inspired and enlightened us. Henrik Blum's influence on our thinking is tremendous, as it is for many other students who have worked with him at the University of California, Berkeley. Dorothy Oda, our faculty partner in community health nursing at the University of California, San Francisco, has been personally supportive throughout the process of writing this book; she also has been incredibly generous in sharing her materials on consultation. Rick Love not only typed most of the manuscript, he even read it and told us when we were not making sense. Hanna Regev typed and read the rest. Their congenial collaboration and support made the final preparation of the manuscript a pleasure. Alison Miller and Suzi Epstein, our editors at Mosby, had faith that we would get the book done, were available when we needed help, and otherwise left us alone to work. Diane Ackermann, our manuscript editor, clarified the presentation of our ideas. Ellen Caulfield, Program Manager, and Lynn Friss, Planner, of the Area Agency on Aging, with whom we did case studies, gave us much assistance. Last but not least, several generations of graduate and undergraduate students in nursing at the University of California, San Francisco who have been in our community health nursing courses have also helped to shape our ideas and experiences. Those who worked with us on the two case studies in Chapters 7 and 8 are individually acknowledged there. To them and to their classmates, past and present, go our thanks.

A special thanks goes to Carole Kelly's husband, Dan, and their two sons, Matthew and Michael, who throughout the entire process were interested, understanding, and encouraging. With their help a semblance of normal family life was made possible.

CONTENTS

1

SYSTEMS AND HOLISM

This book is about the collaboration of human service workers with communities and aggregates to plan and evaluate health and human services. Thus we are concerned with people who are continuously interacting with their natural, physical, and psychosocial environments as we work together to bring about desired change. Since we also stress that this collaboration is an orderly process, we need a framework to help us all understand communities so that we can work with the complex relationships and interactions of people in and among communities without losing sight of the integrity of the whole community. The authors believe, then, that systems theory, systems analysis, and holism provide a framework to guide not only the understanding of community systems but also the collaboration of human service workers with them. In this chapter we discuss the historical background of general systems theory, the key properties and concepts of human systems, and the systems-based model of collaborative processes for community change.

The term *systems* and systems terminology in general are not only pervasive in a variety of physical and human sciences but have become part of common everyday language as in "all systems are go" and "I got feedback on the proposal." Our interest in systems is not new, since systems have been studied for centuries. The definition of *systems* is derived from the Greek words, *systema*, meaning a whole compounded of parts and *synistanai*, meaning to come together.[1]

We use and understand the term *system* in basically two ways. In the first, *system* is the organized whole or the set of interacting elements.[2] In other words, *system* refers to the entity or object of interest. Thus we often refer to individuals, families, communities, and organizations as systems. In the second sense, *system* is the method or set of procedures governing how objects are organized.[1] For example, libraries use the Dewey decimal system for organizing books. In health and human services, systems analysis and systems engineering are management and decision-making processes that are used in complex organizations.

These two meanings of *system* are complementary, not contradictory. They reflect different points of reference and emphasis in developing and using knowledge about what systems are and how they work. Both meanings and uses are grounded in general systems theory, the overriding theoretical framework for many kinds of special systems in a variety of disciplines and practice arenas.

HISTORY

When von Bertalanffy,[3] a biologist, introduced his ideas in the mid-1950s, he broke with traditional scientific thought. He advocated a theoretical approach to the study of living systems that deviated from the prevailing mechanistic school of thought, which up until then had dominated scientific endeavors in all disciplines. As a result of his work in theoretical biology, he became convinced that many of the areas for investigation in the biological, behavioral, and social sciences that deal with the self-regulation and the purposive organization of living systems could not be addressed by and did not even enter into classical physical science considerations.

In the Newtonian mechanistic world view, the model for any living and nonliving system is a machine composed of identifiable elementary parts. Since the objects of analysis are these elementary static parts, the mode of analysis is reductionistic, requiring breaking the system down into its most basic parts and searching for the objectively measurable causal relationships between these parts.[4] The ultimate aim of this kind of analysis is to predict with a high level of accuracy the nature of the whole based on an understanding of the individual parts that when added together constitute the whole. In other words, the whole is equal to the sum of its parts, so one seeks to understand the whole system by analyzing its component parts and adding those analyses together. For example, human service workers are being reductionistic in assessing community health when we focus only on physical health factors and do not consider measuring the interrelated psychological, social, and environmental factors. Because the reductionistic approach is basic to the "hard" or physical sciences, objective measures, quantitative data, and experimental designs that include strict control and the manipulation of variables by the investigator predominate in the research methods in these disciplines.

This reductionistic model works fine when one is talking about automobile engines or relatively closed systems with well-defined boundaries that isolate them from external forces and parts that interact in a fixed, predetermined manner.[5] The machine model does not work well when one applies it to open living systems such as individuals, communities, or organizations. Such systems are not isolated from external forces and are capable of self-transformation in response to external influences that they cannot control or manipulate. The reductionistic model cannot adequately deal with this self-transformation; another model is needed.

To meet this need, von Bertalanffy proposed an organismic model based in Einstein's theory and in quantum physics. This organismic view of a complex living system is based on the assumption that the whole is more than the mere sum of its parts. The characteristics of the system as a whole are different from and therefore not reducible to the characteristics of its parts. The object of analysis is the system as a whole. Understanding the functioning of the whole system cannot be achieved through an analysis of its parts and from their context and if they are treated in isolation of each other. Holistic analysis must take into account not only the interrelationships of the parts but also the parts in relation to the whole. Parts are still of interest but primarily in terms of how they fit together and contribute to the way the system works as a whole.[4]

An organismic or holistic approach to systems analysis, in our case assessment, planning, change, and evaluation, influences what kind of data are gathered, how they are gathered, and how they are used to make decisions. Its methods include multidimensional measures, the gathering of subjective qualitative data through interview and observation in naturalistic settings, quasi-experimental designs in which all the variables cannot be controlled, and recognition of the influence of the observer on the observed.

The organismic view is not a replacement for the mechanistic view. Instead it provides a way to more fully understand the nature of open human systems that cannot be adequately explained by the mechanistic model. Both views focus on systems, but systems of different types. Both views provide valuable information about systems even though they focus on different aspects of those systems. In the study of all systems, the elementary parts, which are the fundamental reality for the mechanistic disciplines, are isolated for detailed analysis, but they cannot be fully understood without reference to their organized whole, which is accomplished through the holistic fields.

General systems theory emerged to serve as the umbrella framework, linking these two seemingly divergent views of systems together. General systems theory provides a common language that is applicable to systems of *all* types whether in physics, chemistry, biology, psychology, sociology, economics, or management sciences. Therefore, general systems theory is often referred to as a supradiscipline, the aim of which is to maximize the theoretical achievements in the study of systems by improving communication and sharing knowledge among specialists in different fields.[6]

PROPERTIES OF SYSTEMS

The unifying language of general systems theory describes the macroscopic properties that are characteristic of all systems to varying degrees. The whole system demonstrates these macroscopic properties because of its organization and integrated functioning.[7] Variations in the degree to which systems manifest these properties are reflected in the way in which they are specifically defined for each special type of system. For example, the property of wholeness of a closed system is more appropriately defined as equal to the sum of its parts, whereas in an open system, wholeness is described as more than and different from the sum of its parts. In addition to wholeness, these properties are openness, interdependence, hierarchical organization,

---

GENERAL SYSTEMS THEORY OVERVIEW*

SELECTED CONTRIBUTORS

Philosophy
   E. Laszlo, L. von Bertalanffy, J. Sutherland
Mechanistic theory
   Cybernetics: N. Wiener, R. Ashby
   Game theory: O. Morgerstern, J. von Neumann
   Information theory: C. Shannon, W. Weaver
Organismic theory
   Biology: L. von Bertalanffy, J. Miller, A. Rapport
   Psychiatry: W. Gray, N. Rizzo
   Sociology: W. Buckley, T. Parsons
   Economics: K. Boulding
Systems analysis
   Management/operations research: R. Ackoff, C.W. Churchman, G. Vickers
   Engineering: A.D. Hall, R.E. Fagen

KEY PROPERTIES OF SYSTEM CONSTRUCT

Openness: boundary, energy, environment, input, negentropy, output, throughput
Wholeness: nonsummativity
Interdependence: centralization, segregation, systematization
Hierarchy: organization, subsystem, suprasystem
Self-regulation: feedback, optimization, suboptimization
Dynamic activity: equilibrium, homeostasis, morphogenesis, morphostasis, steady state
Goal directedness: equifinality

Modified from Bisch, S.: General systems theory overview, Unpublished paper, 1981.
*For further information about these systems theories, the reader is referred to the bibliography at the end of the book.

self-regulation, dynamic activity, and goal directedness.[8,9] This list of properties also provides a way to organize the vast array of concepts that are used to describe the structure and functions of all systems. The box above illustrates an approach to this kind of organization. For the purposes of our discussion of these characteristics, we must artificially separate them when in actuality they, like the systems they describe, are so interrelated that no one property can be clearly defined and understood without reference to all the others.

Our discussion of these broadly defined properties of systems focuses on the organismic holistic view, since we are most concerned with complex open living systems such as communities, aggregates, and organizations.

Openness

The degree of openness of a system is determined by the system's interaction with its surrounding environment. The environment is everything outside of the system that affects and is affected by the system. An open system continuously exchanges resources with its environment across its boundary, which is the line of demarcation separating the system from its environment. The system's boundary helps to maintain the system's integrity and acts as a filter to monitor the flow of resources in and out of the system.[10]

Openness is critical to the continual viability of living systems. A system receives input in the form of matter, energy, and information from its environment and through its internal processes, called throughput, converts the input into output, which is released into its environment. The system's output may modify the input required for its functioning through feedback or may become input for other systems in the environment. This exchange, which provides free replenishable energy for the work of the system, enables the system to maintain as well as to transform itself. In Chapter 2, we discuss a system's maintenance and transformation as first- and second-order change respectively. Open systems are considered negentropic because they have free energy available for the system's operations and have the capacity to progress toward greater complexity and order. Closed systems, because of little or no exchange with their environments, progress toward disorder and decay.[10]

Sometimes for purposes of studying a complex system, analysts will close the system or a part of it, that is, a subsystem, by setting an artificial boundary around the parts to be studied and will treat the system as independent of its surrounding environment. This allows the analysts to focus only on what occurs within the subsystem of interest and temporarily to ignore any external influences. This example is not a realistic representation, but it does allow the analysts to study a part of the total system as a preliminary step in considering the greater complexity of the total open system.[11] However, the analysts must bear in mind that their understanding of the subsystem of interest will be different when they consider it in the context of the total system.

Wholeness

It is necessary to begin this discussion of the property of wholeness with a description of holism because the meaning of wholeness cannot be understood without reference to the philosophical premises of holism. It is also useful to preface this more detailed discussion of the properties of a system with a discussion of its philosophical origins. In fact, general systems theory is often viewed as the attempt to merge the intuitive skills of the philosopher with the instrumental skills of the scientist.[5]

It is not surprising that the term *holism*, a derivation of the Greek word *holos*, meaning whole, was first used by a man who had great interest in both philosophy and biology. In 1926, Jan Smuts stated his belief in the existence of a synthetic tendency in the universe to ultimately interconnect everything. This synthesizing process, which he referred to as holism, leads to the evolution of a progressive series of greater wholes. Wholeness, then, is a fundamental characteristic of nature.[12]

Smuts is credited with being first to use holism to describe this tendency for universal interconnectedness in Western thought, but the idea of interconnectedness existed long before that in the Eastern world.

> For the Eastern mystic, all things and events perceived by the senses are interrelated, connected, and are but different aspects or manifestations of the same ultimate reality. Our tendency to divide the perceived world into individual and separate things and to experience ourselves as isolated egos in this world is seen as an illusion which comes from our measuring and categorizing mentality.[13]

The unity and perpetual motion of nature are basic elements in Eastern mystical thinking.

It is only with the advent of quantum theory that this interconnectedness of nature, which was intuitively known by the Eastern mystic and the Western philosopher, has been given scientific validity. Experiments have shown that particles affect each other regardless of the distance between them. The interaction is so complete that cause and effect cannot be separated. In fact, "a single variable can be both cause and effect."[14] Heisenberg extended this notion of interconnectedness to encompass the way nature is studied. He proposed that objects are changed in the process of being studied, so that every observation is different because of the interaction between observer and observed. Human beings are an integral part of nature and cannot stand outside of nature to observe and measure it.[15] Thus there is a notion of unbroken wholeness: the continual dynamic relationships of parts to parts and parts to whole that extend from atoms to the entire universe. Systems as wholes can be analyzed in different ways by different observers, providing equally valid information. Modern physicists are saying that holism, instability, and variability are fundamental principles on the basis of which our thinking must be reoriented.[16]

Holistic thinking has precipitated changes in health care delivery in the United States by creating a model of care that competes with the pervasive medical model. Table 1-1 summarizes some of the primary differences between the medical model, which is based on the mechanistic systems view, and the holistic health model, which is based on the organismic systems view. As a result of the emerging holistic approaches to health care, alternate services now exist that value whole persons and their right to assume active responsibility for and participation in making and implementing decisions that affect their current and future health states.

Holistic health care approaches such as meditation, visualization, biofeedback, polarity therapy, and homeopathy are primarily directed toward the individual or family in the context of their environments or as part of the greater community system. These individually oriented holistic approaches are not applicable to the whole community as client. Community-oriented holistic approaches are directed toward maximizing total community health and wholeness. Community health must then be viewed as more than the sum of the health states of its individual members.[17]

TABLE 1-1

Comparison of selected characteristics of medical and holistic health models

Medical model	Holistic health model
Disease focused	Whole-client focused (person-community)
Based on mind-body dualism, reductionistic germ theory, and Newtonian physics	Based on organismic, holistic, and ecological theories and quantum physics
Discrete causation	Multiple interacting influences
Patient involuntarily assaulted by disease-causing agents	Shared personal and societal responsibility for illness
Chemical and physical intervention to counteract causal effects	Multiple interventions directed at individual, institutional, and societal levels
Disease treated by technically competent specialist	Collaboration on interventions with multiple practitioners
Patient must comply with prescriptions of specialist	Client (person-community) is the ultimate decision maker
Emphasis on alleviating symptoms and curing disease	Emphasis on maximizing health and wholeness

Modified from Donnelley, G.F., and others: The nursing system: issues, ethics, and politics, New York, 1980, John Wiley & Sons, Inc. p. 205; data also from Hays-Bautista, D., and Harveston, D.S.: Holistic health care, Social Policy 7:7-13, March-April 1977.

The modifications in Table 1-1 expand the holistic health model so that it is applicable to the community system as the client.

Holistic approaches require us as human service workers to reorient our thinking about how we conceptualize community health and how we interact and collaborate with communities. Cottrell and Goeppinger[18,19] refer to evolving ways to describe and measure community competence. The way we as consultants conceptualize communities also influences the questions they ask about them and the kinds of data we gather to address those questions. Some approaches to data collection and analysis are discussed in Chapters 5 and 6.

Holism and the interconnectedness of living systems suggest that the wholeness of a system must be defined as a synthesis rather than as a summation of its parts and that the process is synergistic rather than additive. Thus as previously defined, the whole is more than and therefore different from the sum of its parts. The parts of the whole are dynamically interrelated, but it is the totality of the organization of its interrelated parts that determines the unique characteristics of the whole, which cannot be created by simply adding the parts together. In other words, the whole does not exist simply by virtue of its parts but has a character and life of its own because it has additional properties of pattern and organization that emerge as a result of the interrelationships of its parts.[20] For example, hydrogen and oxygen combine to form water, whose properties in no way reflect the properties of either hydrogen or oxygen. The authors believe that the quality of the ideas and their presentation in this book are better because they are the synthesis of our ideas. The product is vastly superior to what any one of us could have produced.

The examples illustrate another aspect of wholeness. The properties of the whole cannot be understood by analyzing parts of the whole separately and independently of each other. One achieves understanding of the parts in this way but cannot get an adequate picture of reality because parts are not isolated but rather are integral parts of the whole they create. The whole and its parts cannot be understood without reference to each other.[21]

To understand a system as a whole, one must consider its parts in relation to its parts, its parts in relation to the whole, and the whole in relation to the parts. When a community is viewed as a whole system, the interrelationships among its citizens and institutions, how they fit together and work together to create the pattern and organization of the community—its norms, values, and decision and action styles—as well as how the community's pattern and organization influences the functioning and interrelationships of its citizens and institutions must be examined. However, this is only part of the interconnectedness, as can be seen in the discussion of the interaction of the whole system with other whole systems in the section on hierarchical organization.

Interdependence

Interdependence refers to the nature of the relationships, the interactions, and the interconnections within and among systems. Because of the fundamental interconnectedness of the universe, this property extends not only to the relationships among the parts within systems but also to the relationships among the systems in the hierarchical order of the universe. For simplicity's sake, we will restrict the discussion of interdependence here to the internal relationships of a system and will discuss interdependence among systems in the section on hierarchical organization.

Parts of a system are interdependently interrelated in such a way that change in one part of the system ripples or reverberates throughout the entire system. This ripple effect precipitates change in other *parts* of the system and therefore in the *whole* system. It is this interdependent functioning of the parts that creates the wholeness of the system so that the system behaves as a whole single entity and not as a mere conglomeration of individual parts.[22,23]

Wholeness and interdependence are related properties, since the former depends in part on the latter. More specifically, it is the degree of interdependence of the parts of a system that determines the degree of wholeness of the system.[23] For example, in discussing the use of a holistic systems approach to planning and evaluation with aggregates and communities, we are considering both as systems even though a community may exhibit a greater degree of wholeness, particularly if it is an ethnic community with strongly tied families living within the same geographical boundary, as compared to an aggregate of elderly clients who regularly attend senior citizens dining sites. In both the ethnic community and the elderly aggregate there are interdependent relationships and common interests that tie them together. However, the relationships and ties may be stronger in the ethnic community, which means that as a system it exhibits greater interdependence and complexity. Both are systems with properties of interdependence and wholeness and can therefore be approached from a holistic perspective. The difference is a matter of degree.

Wholeness and interdependence are not absolute. By this we mean that the parts of a system are not usually locked into such permanent arrangements that change in these arrangements is impossible.[24] In fact, the transitory nature of interdependent relationships creates the potential for change in the whole system. We discuss this transformation potential in the section on dynamic activity.

System concepts organize the shifts in arrangements and formations of new alignments that occur within systems into three types. *Progressive systematization* refers to the process of change in the interrelationships of parts of the system toward increasing interdependence. This process involves the strengthening of existing relationships, the establishment of new relationships among parts that were previously unrelated, and the addition of new parts and relationships to the system. The end result is an increase in the complexity of the network of the system's relationships toward greater unity and coherence of the whole system.[25] Communities may undergo progressive systematization when they are faced with a threat from their external environment. An example is a government proposal to create a toxic waste disposal site within the community's watershed. Such an external threat could galvanize the community's many subsystems into concerted action in opposition to the proposal.

Opposite to progressive systematization is *progressive segregation,* in which the existing relationships are weakened or severed and new relationships are not established. Thus parts of the system become unrelated or tenuously related to other parts and may function more independently. If this segregation process continues, it can lead to decay of the total system so that the system functions chaotically or no longer functions as a unified whole. Another possible end result is that the organization of the system changes in the direction of increasing subdivision so that instead of breaking apart, the system becomes composed of subsystems that are still interrelated but have differentiated functions. The system not only survives but increases its complexity and enhances its functioning.[23] Progressive segregation is occurring in some communities where agencies that previously had a relatively predictable categorical federal funding base are now being forced to compete with each other for block-grant funds. This phenomenon has been destructive to the functioning of these community agencies as a relatively unified whole.

Both systematization and segregation can occur simultaneously. A system can enlarge itself by adding new parts and relationships and thereby increase its complexity. It manages its growth by differentiating its functioning and thereby continues to exist.[25]

The third type of realignment is *centralization,* in which one part of the system takes on the key role in the functioning of the system. It is called the leading part, and all the other parts of the system are centered around it. Because of its importance to the system, a minor change in the leading part can cause considerable reverberation and change throughout the system and in the whole system itself. Centralization can accompany either systematization or segregation because both processes can be controlled by the leading part.[25] State-level agencies that are designated to apportion health service block-grant funds have achieved a centralization in the state government system greater than many of them have enjoyed before.

Hierarchical organization

This characteristic of systems means that open living systems are interrelated in an organized fashion and do not exist in random association with each other. We already mentioned in the section on wholeness that the synthetic tendency in the universe drives it toward increasing complexity and wholeness. Therefore systems exist in a ranked order or hierarchy of increasing levels of complexity. In terms of the species *Homo sapiens,* this hierarchy ranges from subatomic particles at the lowest end, through molecules, cells, organs, persons, families, aggregates, organizations, communities, and societies to the biosphere and beyond at the highest end. There is no judgment about the intrinsic value or worth involved in the ranking.[26] A system at a higher level of complexity, such as a community, is not more important than a system at a lower level of complexity, such as an aggregate; the community is just more complex.

We have been referring to a system as a synthesis of its parts. It is more descriptive to refer to its parts as subsystems so that a system is a synthesis of its own subsystems. However, the system itself is a subsystem of its own higher level system or suprasystem. In this way a system's parts can also be conceptualized as systems, albeit lower level, less complex ones. A helpful analogy may be a box, within a box, within a box, and so forth. We conceptualized communities and aggregates as systems when we discussed interdependence. Because of the hierarchical organization of systems, they are not separate isolated systems but are interrelated ones. In our case study, the elderly aggregate is only one subsystem of the greater system or suprasystem of the community.

Hierarchical organization also means that one must consider a system within its context. Attention may be focused at one level, but one must be aware of the influence of other systems at higher and lower levels. If a community human service worker is working with a family, she or he knows that its functioning as a family system is influenced by the interactions and communications among its individual members. The worker must also recognize that the nature of the local community and society of which the family is a subsystem also influence the family's functioning. The local community norms and values and laws of a society even determine what is accepted family size and composition.

Because of the interconnectedness of systems and the flow of information and resources among systems up and down the hierarchy, the ripple effect that we talk about occurring within systems also occurs among systems. In other words, change at all levels of the hierarchy of systems eventually spreads throughout the hierarchy. Influences and fluctuations at one level come from and are felt at the immediate higher and lower levels as well as at distally related levels.

Hierarchical organization has important implications not only for one's understanding of systems but also for planning and evaluating changes in systems. One must look for possible ways to bring about change at various levels in the hierarchy and to assess and evaluate their impact at different hierarchical levels.[26] For example, change in the level and distribution of the federal budget's expenditures for health and human services has caused ripple effects, tidal waves in some areas, throughout the nation.

Self-regulation

This property refers to the ability of the system to continually guide its own activity to ensure that the system attains its purpose or goals. The end result of this cybernation may be maintenance of the system's existing form over time *in spite of* internal and external forces that precipitate disturbances and fluctuations, or transformations of its existing form into a new form *because of* the disturbances and fluctuations.[27] Self-regulation may in fact be a misnomer because it conveys the idea of maintenance. Self-transformation may be a more descriptive concept particularly for living systems. The self-transformation capability of complex open systems is discussed in the section on dynamic activity.

Self-regulation is possible because of the feedback mechanism for monitoring the flow of information between the system and its environment (external feedback) and among the subsystems of the system (internal feedback). The information on the system's performance that is received by the system is used to adjust the quality and nature of internal processes and its future input.[28] The feedback mechanism is the same for internal and external feedback, but for ease of discussion the external feedback is our point of reference.

In other words, the output or products of the system's operations that are released into the system's environment provide information about its outcomes in its environment. The outcomes affect the other systems as intended or unintended consequences of the system's activities. The system monitors the environmental responses to its output and adjusts itself accordingly by modifying its subsystems and altering its boundary's permeability.[28]

When people are trying to change their behavior, for example, going on a diet to lose weight, they seek feedback on how they are doing. They may weigh themselves at regular intervals, obtain diet counseling, attend exercise classes, and so on. They use the information that they receive as a result of these efforts to adjust their activities, depending on how successfully they are progressing in achieving their desired weight loss or smaller clothes sizes.

In Chapter 5 we describe the component of evaluation that focuses on assessing the impact or consequences of a program or other activity on its community. The data so obtained are feedback to the decision-makers to guide their choices about the value and continuation of the program or activity.

There are two types of feedback. The first is negative feedback, in which information is fed back into the system to correct or decrease its deviations from the system's expected performance, which is necessary to maintain its steady state. Changes occur in the system's input and processes but do so within predetermined limits to perpetuate the system's existing structure and function. Positive feedback increases rather than decreases deviations from the system's steady-state performance. It precipitates considerable change in the system's input and processes to the extent that the system's existing steady state is destroyed, and if unchecked, it can lead to the self-destruction of the whole system. However, positive feedback is not necessarily detrimental because it can enhance the system's capability to grow and develop and become more complex. A system's existing structure may need to be altered and even destroyed in the process of transformation to new and more complex structures.[10] In a sense, the system undergoes a crisis, which is also an opportunity for growth.

The limits on the quantity and quality of the system's self-regulated changes toward maintenance or transformation vary from system to system and over time. Human beings in early embryonic stages undergo considerable transformation when they progress in complexity from fertilized ova to fetuses. However, in later adult developmental stages, the possible transformations are restricted by the limits of the human system.

Complex systems, such as a community, also have transformation limits in the form of implicit rules, sociocultural values, and laws on the basis of which individual citizens and institutions detect and take action to correct deviations and control the community's steady state. In fact, unlike human beings, a community's limits are more flexible and more subject to change. A community, then, has greater potential than human beings to change its overall structure. This is second-order change, which we discuss in Chapter 2.

We have been talking about feedback, which provides only existing contextual information on the system's performance. Reeves adds *feedforward* to describe the information about the future conditions and contexts in which the system will be functioning interdependently. To help a community system to achieve its desired futures and goals (see Chapter 2), one must attempt to anticipate the future context of the community and under what conditions it will be functioning so as to anticipate the adjustments that may be necessary to help the community achieve its goals.[29]

Finally, optimization is another way to describe a system's ability to guide its actions. It involves altering the system's operations to enable it to concentrate its efforts on a particular activity or in a specific subsystem to achieve the best possible outcomes. This selective attention may be mandated by the needs and desires of the whole system, but there are opportunity costs in that resources that are devoted to one subsystem or set of activities cannot be used elsewhere or for other purposes. "Optimizing one subsystem results in sub-optimizing all the rest."[30] Given a fixed budget, a community that elects to optimize its police force for citizen protection must suboptimize all other community services.

Dynamic activity

Dynamic activity, as the term implies, means that systems are active, not static. "Flowing wholeness . . . highly organized but always in process."[31] A system's properties affect the ability of the system to stay in perpetual motion even if it appears to be standing still. However, the kind of activity is not described in the same way for all systems.

Buckley argues that the mechanistic-equilibrium model is not appropriate for open living systems, particularly complex societal systems.[32] Equilibrium, a relatively fixed state of balance among the forces operating in and on systems, is more descriptive of relatively closed systems that have no internal processes for change.[33] Since such systems have no exchange with their environments to replenish energy, the equilibrium they achieve is "not a healthy balance . . . (but) a kind of death."[14]

Buckley prefers steady state, homeostasis, or its variant, homeokinesis, to refer to open systems that have the capacity for self-regulation. However, the changes that homeostatic systems make are primarily adjustments to environmental input and feedback and are geared to structural maintenance.[34]

He proposes that complex adaptive systems, like sociocultural systems organizations, have internal capacities for change. They are "open internally as well as externally in that interchanges among their components may result in significant changes in the nature of the components themselves with important consequences for the system as a whole."[34] Complex adaptive systems have processes for self-maintenance, which Buckley called *morphostasis,* but more importantly, systems have processes for self-transformation, called *morphogenesis.* Self-directed changes or the elaboration of the structures of systems are the means for survival in a rapidly changing environment. If complex adaptive systems have the capacity for self-transformation, it may then be less valid to attribute permanence to their structures and to assume that the overall structure of such systems determines their functions. The more appropriate question may be "how is structure created, maintained, and re-created?"[35]

Prigogine provides the theoretical basis for Buckley's suppositions. In 1977, he won the Nobel Prize for Chemistry for his theory of dissipative structures, which describes and explains the irreversible processes in nature that enable whole living systems to transform themselves.[12] Before he proposed his theory, the predominant use of the mechanistic-equilibrium model meant that living systems had to be viewed as machines without the internal capacity to refuel and regenerate themselves over time and as entropic systems because they progress toward maximum disorder and eventual decay. This view did not allow for the explanation of the reality that living systems, particularly complex ones, can and do evolve into higher orders of complexity throughout their lifetimes.[36]

Prigogine stated in his theory that an open living system is a complex dissipative structure that requires a tremendous amount of energy to maintain all its complex interconnections and its structural integrity. In a dissipative structure, instead of the energy being bound up in maintaining a deadly equilibrium as it is in closed systems, the system dissipates or dumps this energy into its surrounding environment and is able to take in new energy to replenish its supplies. A dissipative structure also maintains a steady state, but in contrast to equilibrium systems, this constancy is maintained in a continuous flow of energy. This continuous movement of energy within and throughout the system creates the potential for considerable internal fluctuations. Systems that are highly complex are also highly unstable. Because of this high instability, they are also susceptible to considerable change and transformation. If the internal fluctuations reach critical proportion, they perturb the system and shake up the old connections, thereby enabling the system to create new connections and to reorganize itself into a new whole with a character that is different from the old one.[14,36]

Goal directedness

All the activity of the system occurs in a coherent rather than a random fashion because the system's parts are working together to achieve some overriding goal or purpose of the system in interaction with the environment. However, in open living systems goals or purpose are not totally fixed and unchanging. The purpose is determined by the initial conditions at the creation of the system, but this initial purpose is not necessarily the final one that is achieved.

Systems are characterized by equifinality, in which the same end state is reached from a number of starting points. Because of the exchange of resources of an open living system and its dynamic activity, a system can achieve an end state that is relatively independent of its starting conditions and is determined only by the limits of the system in interaction with its environment.[37] The end result is relatively unpredictable. For example, in times of relatively plentiful funding and other resources, communities can pursue many goals through the establishment of numerous programs. When resources become scarcer, goals must be subjected to priority analysis and some programs are reduced or eliminated.

Summary

General systems theory provides the human service worker with a set of concepts for both the structural and functional analyses of community and aggregates as whole systems. Structural concepts describe aggregates as subsystems in interdependent relations with all other subsystems within the geopolitical boundaries of the community system and the community system in interdependent relations with all other suprasystems in its surrounding environment. Functional concepts describe a community system as an open adaptive system and therefore constantly exchanging information and resources internally among its subsystems and externally with other systems in its environment, as a system in a state of goal-directed dynamic activity in which change in one part of the system or on its environment ripples throughout; and as a system capable of self-regulation and self-direction not only for self-maintenance, but for self-transformation as well.

A MODEL OF COLLABORATION IN CHANGE

We as human service workers or consultants need a framework, a set of concepts and values for collaborative work with communities and aggregates, to help in comprehending what we see and experience and to guide what we do. Without a framework, consultants would have difficulty organizing and understanding community work. Too rigid or narrow a framework would limit our view. Too broad a framework would provide no direction at all. The model presented on p. 16 is based in general systems theory and is a framework whose components are general enough to have broad applicability.[38] This generality is purposive to ensure that the model can be used in many circumstances.

Fig. 1 illustrates the use of systems concepts to describe a collaborative process for change. The two overlapping circles represent the participant systems in the change process, namely, the consultant system and the community/aggregate target system. Both are viewed as open systems whose boundaries permit the free exchange of resources with each other and with their environments. Each of these systems is composed of a hierarchical order of subsystems and suprasystems (represented by the concentric circles).

For example, in the case study of the *Senior resources survey* (see Chapter 7) the consultant system is composed of several subsystems: the community health nursing faculty, community health nursing students, and members of the Nursing Dynamics Corporation (NDC). Suprasystems include NDC and the School of Nursing. The community system is composed of the County Area Agency on Aging, the Commis-

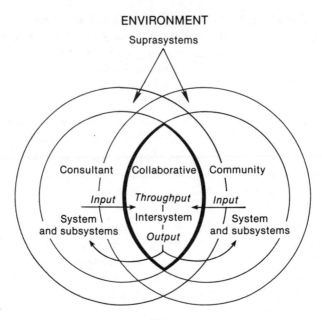

FIG. 1
Model of collaboration in change.

sion on Aging, and agencies in the county that offered services to the elderly population; each of these is a subsystem. Community suprasystems include the State Department of Aging and the United States government, which administers the Older
Americans Act.

The primary focus of the model is the intersystem, a conceptualization borrowed
from Chin,[33] which is the arena in which the two systems interact.[39] Since the
consultant and community systems are not the main focus of the model, their
boundaries are drawn lightly. Essentially they are part of the intersystem's environment.

There are several advantages to this arrangement of the circles that represent the
key systems. The first is that the model highlights that the desired change is not
planned by outsiders alone, working from outside of the community target system,
nor by insiders alone, working from inside the community target system, but rather
by both consultant and participants in the community system working together within a collaborative intersystem. Consultants and community participants jointly assume the change-agent role[40] and participate equally in the creation of a new third
system, which has a life of its own and whose character is necessarily different from
those of both the consultant and the community systems.

According to the way the model is drawn, it gives the impression that consultants
participate in the collaborative intersystem as members of a consultant system that

originally is not part of the community system. This portrayal implies that the prospective consultants have had no previous ties or relationships with the community system. We know that in reality the original positions of the consultant and community systems vis-a-vis each other are often blurred. A prime example are our case studies in which the NDC and faculty members of the consultant system who became part of the collaborative intersystem were and continued to be active members of the community system. Because of these blurred positions, consultants often have insider and outsider views of the target system simultaneously. Some of the advantages and disadvantages of this dual view are summarized in Chapter 5.

The authors believe that the conceptualization of an intersystem in which collaborative planning for change takes place resolves some of the dilemmas inherent in the change models of other systems.[33] These models require that the change agent be an insider or, if an outsider, attempt to become part of the community target system to effectively contribute to bringing about community change. In our model, the consultants and the community members are neither outsiders nor insiders, but all are participants in all activities in the collaborative intersystem.

The model also clearly demonstrates the interdependence of all systems so that changes in the consultant system, the community system, and other suprasystems in their environments are felt in the collaborative intersystem and vice versa. The participants in the collaborative intersystem do not sacrifice their relationships with their respective systems but rather remain interdependent parts in them. These linkages are essential so that community participants have continual input and feedback from their constituencies. Consultants also need connections with their own reference groups for support and feedback.

Consultant and community participants contribute their own input to the collaborative intersystem. This input is, in part, determined by the nature of their respective systems. Consultants, as part of organizations or agencies, may provide financial, material, and manpower resources. They also provide input in the less tangible forms of knowledge and skills required for the specific purpose of the consultation. This theoretical expertise and practical experience may be in specialized content areas such as environmental protection and rehabilitation or generalized process areas such as management, community organization, and evaluation. Consultants also bring attitudes and skills that affect the way the collaborative consultation process is carried out to achieve desired goals. These include the consultant's flexibility, adaptability, interpersonal and communication skills, cultural sensitivity, set of ground rules for working relationships, and so on. Community participants contribute similar kinds of input, perhaps less in terms of financial and material resources, but certainly in terms of manpower, knowledge, and skills pertaining to their unique situation. The latter factors are essential input, since community participants have knowledge of their own wants, needs, and the working of their systems that outsiders can never acquire. Input does not necessarily remain the same throughout the collaborative process. The kind, quality, and quantity of input vary as circumstances change.

Through the collaboration of the consultant and community participants, input is conveted into plans and programs as a means to attain the desired goals. Chapter 7 is devoted to discussing these processes and some of the kinds of changes that result.

The model also points out that the output of the collaborative intersystem has consequences not only for the community system but also for the consultant system as well as their subsystems and suprasystems. These consequences may be in terms of new programs, parks, or public transit systems. They may also be in the less tangible form of having learned something, having gained knowledge and experience, and having been changed as a result. Tangible output of the *Needs and Life-Style Assessment* described in Chapter 7 include the development of some programs for the elderly and changes in some existing ones. Intangible consequences changed the evaluators; we learned a great deal about assessment and a lot about ourselves as well.

A pervasive feature of the model is change: change that is mutual and dynamic. The ultimate goal of the collaborative process is to bring about the target system's desired change. But in the process of achieving this goal, all participants also experience change because of their experience in the collaborative intersystem, as they receive inputs and feedback from their respective systems, as they are influenced by their environments, and as they live with the consequences of their collaborative efforts. Change is not only apparent in the outcomes at the end of the process but also, in terms of the measured differences in the target system, is part of the process throughout its course. Change in people and in the systems in which they interact is necessary to bring about whatever change people and their systems desire. Change is not only constant, it is all pervading.

REFERENCES

1. Webster's Third New International Dictionary of the English Language (unabridged), Springfield, Mass., 1981, G & C Merriam Co.
2. von Bertalanffy, L.V.: Perspectives on general systems theory, New York, 1975, George Braziller, Inc.
3. von Bertalanffy, L.V.: General systems theory: a critical review. In Buckley, W., editor: Modern systems research for the behavioral sciences, Chicago, 1968, Aldine Publishing Co., pp. 11-30.
4. Ritterman, M.K.: Paradigmatic classification of family therapy theories, Family Process **16**:26-48, March 1977.
5. Sutherland, J.W.: A general systems philosophy for the social and behavioral sciences, New York, 1973, George Braziller, Inc., pp. 19-51.
6. Sutherland, p. 19.
7. Bunge, M.: A systems concept of society: beyond individualism and holism, General Systems Yearbook **24**:27-44, 1979.
8. Battista, J.R.: The holistic paradigm and general systems theory, General Systems Yearbook **22**:65-71, 1977.

9. Hall, A.D., and Fagen, R.E.: Definition of system. In Buckley, W., editor: Modern systems research for the behavioral sciences, Chicago, 1968, Aldine Publishing Co., pp. 81-92.
10. Hazzard, M.E.: An overview of systems theory, Nursing Clinics of North America **6**:385-393, 1971.
11. Reeves, P.N., Bergwall, D.E., and Woodside, N.B.: Introduction to health planning, ed. 2, Washington, D.C., 1979, Information Resources Press, pp. 41-57.
12. Flynn, P.A.: Holistic health: the art and science of care, Bowie, Md., 1980, Robert J. Brady Co., pp. 1-13.
13. Capra, F.: The tau of physics, New York, 1975, Banton Books, p. 10.
14. Ferguson, M.: The aquarian conspiracy: personal and social transformations in the 1980s, Los Angeles, 1980, J.P. Tarcher Inc., p. 157.
15. Flynn, pp. 2-4.
16. Blattner, B.: Holistic nursing, Englewood Cliffs, N.J., 1981, Prentice-Hall, Inc.
17. The definition and role of public health nursing practice in the delivery of health care, American Journal of Public Health **72**:210-212, February 1982.
18. Cottrell, L.S., Jr.: The competent community. In Kaplan, B.H., Wilson, R.N., and Leighton, A.H., editors: Future elaborations in social psychiatry, New York, 1976, Basic Books, pp. 198-205.
19. Goeppinger, J., and others: Community health is competence, Nursing Outlook **30**:464-467, 1982.
20. Flynn, p. 12.
21. Sutherland, pp. 34-42.
22. Archer, S.E.: Selected community health processes. In Archer, S.E., and Fleshman, R.P.: Community health nursing: patterns and practices, ed. 2, North Sutuate, Mass., 1979, Duxbury Press, pp. 86-88.
23. Hall and Fagen, p. 85.
24. Foster, G.M., and Anderson, B.G.: Medical anthropology, New York, 1978, John Wiley & Sons, pp. 11-12.
25. Hall and Fagen, p. 86.
26. Brody, H., and Sobel, D.S.: A systems view of health and disease, Holistic Health Review **3**:163-178, 1980.
27. Battista, p. 68.
28. Hazzard, p. 391.
29. Reeves and others, pp. 44-45.
30. Archer, S.E., p. 88.
31. Ferguson, M., p. 164.
32. Buckley, W.: Society as a complex adaptive system. In Buckley, W., editor: Modern systems research for the behavioral scientist, Chicago, 1968, Aldine Publishing Co., pp. 490-513.
33. Chin, R.: The utility of systems models and development models for practitioners. In Bennis, W.G., Benne, K.D., Chin, R., and Corey, K.E., editors: The planning of change, New York, 1976, Holt, Rinehart, & Winston, Inc. pp. 90-102.
34. Buckley, W., p. 490.
35. Buckley, W., p. 491.
36. Krieger, D.: Foundations for holistic health nursing practices: the Renaissance nurse, Philadelphia, 1981, J.B. Lippincott, pp. 3-15.
37. von Bertalanffy, 1968, p. 18.

38. Bisch, S.A.: A model for collaboration in change, Unpublished paper, 1981.
39. Foster, G.M.: Applied anthropology, Boston, 1969, Little, Brown, & Co., pp. 115-129.
40. Kerr, G.B.: Rethinking the change agent role in the technical assistance process to facilitate the new international order. In Spitzberg, I., editor: The exchange of expertise: counterparts and the new international order, Boulder, Colo., 1978, Westview Press, pp. 81-97.

2

PLANNING AND CHANGE PROCESSES

Planning and change are inextricably linked, since change or the decision not to change is the outcome of most plans. Because planning and change are major reasons for conducting community and aggregate assessments, human service workers need to be familiar with both of these processes. Assessments are generally a first step in planning for some kind of change. Needs assessments present a clearer picture of a system's baseline data. A comparison of the target aggregate or community system with others like it or with an ideal provides indications of what if any changes are desirable to make the status of the target aggregate or community more like the desired one. Making these kinds of changes involves planning.

PLANNING
Definition

Victor Hugo is said to have observed that man is the only animal that cries because man alone sees the difference between what is and what could be. Were it not for people's abilities to assess reality and to believe in, hope for, and plan for something else, something they believe is better, there would be no need for this book or for others like it. Philosophers reflect on the potential differences between present reality and possible futures. These reflections are essential. People who are action oriented strive to convert these desired futures into reality. Assessment, planning, change, and evaluation are all part of that conversion process.

The planning process has many definitions, almost all of which include the following components:

1. Assessment
2. Diagnosis of needed change
3. Implementation of those changes
4. Evaluation of the outcomes of implementation

Planning also has many definitions. We shall proceed in this discussion with this operational definition of planning: planning is a collaborative, orderly, and cyclic process to attain a mutually agreed-on desired future, or goal. It requires consensus of the participants to implement actions that lead to outcomes, most of which involve change to achieve the goals. Outcomes and their consequences must be evaluated in terms of their contribution to the attainment of the goal. We shall look at each of the concepts in this systems-based definition. From our systems perspective, we also focus our discussion on the community system as a whole, of which the target aggregate in which we are interested is a part. The changes planned for the benefit of the target aggregate must take into account its interdependent relationships with its community system.

Collaborative process. The collaborative process is introduced in Chapter 1 and is discussed from the consultant's perspective and roles in Chapter 4. What we stress here is the need for continuous and active involvement of the people who will be affected by the outcomes of the planning process in all phases of that process. Under this condition, members of the consultant system and members of the target community system work together in a collaborative intersystem throughout the process toward mutually agreed-on goals and outcomes. Implicit in the concept of collaboration is the assumption that consultants and members of the target community share as peers in the collaborative process. Members of each system bring their own values, priorities, ideas, hidden agendas, vested interests, and needs to their shared arena. All must be ready to negotiate compromise, trade off, and otherwise work to achieve the kind of consensus that is essential if the planning process is to be anything more than an exercise in futility and frustration for all concerned. Here again our stress is on collaboration in the planning process between consultants and members of the target community. (See Fig. 1 and the accompanying discussion.)

Collaboration means that consultants and community members in the intersystem together define what is to be done, how, when, by whom, and, most of all, why. In this way both consultants and community members express their preferences and learn from the situations they share and from each other. Collaboration is not characterized by consultants or community members giving each other preconceived lists of goals, alternatives, or actions from which to make choices, nor does it involve forced-choice situations where one must pick one alternative or the other. Rather, collaboration involves all participants in the process who together consider all of the possible options, at least insofar as they can be identified, and share in decision making with the objective of mutual gain.[1] For ease of discussion, we use *collaborative intersystem* and *planning group* interchangeably.

Orderly process. Orderly process addresses the value of planned change, consciously and deliberately brought about through collaboration with members of the community, rather than the creation of chaos. Unfortunately, even the most carefully laid plans for orderly change occasionally backfire, resulting in some degree of chaos and disruption. Although it is not necessarily detrimental to the overall goal of attaining the desired future, chaos has a tendency to get out of hand and to spread far more than participants want. As with many situations and phenomena, chaos should be prevented.

Even though we stress the orderly nature of planning, bear in mind that serendipities can and do occur. These are unexpected and unplanned outcomes that may be more beneficial than the outcomes originally sought. Part of the reason serendipities can occur is that one cannot, even with the aid of computer simulation and other forecasting techniques, anticipate all of the possible alternatives for actions or their consequences. We as planning participants must constantly be alert for the possibility of such happy circumstances and be ready not only to recognize them but also to accept them. Along the same line of thinking, we must also be aware of the possibility of unexpected negative results. In either case, numerous early warning mechanisms to supply timely feedback are essential so that whatever corrections are warranted can be made. Cybernation is as essential in planning as it is in so many other functions.

Cyclic process. Since most of the desired futures that participants in planning agree on are relatively global, attaining them often requires several planning processes over a considerable period of time. Each one of these planning processes should be viewed as a part or segment of a continuing cycle of closely related activities in an ongoing process. Thus one planning activity or process is not discrete from the one that preceded it nor from the one that follows. The final evaluation of outcomes and their consequences in one planning cycle is actually the assessment phase of the next planning cycle. With this conceptualization one plan builds on another and anticipates at least parts of the plans that follow. This process has also been discussed elsewhere.[2-4]

Mutually agreed-on desired future. Collaboration between consultants and community members necessitates sharing and a consensus-achieving approach to all phases of the planning process. Initially and most importantly, participants must reach consensus about what the desired future for the community, of which the target aggregate is a part, should be. This is a normative and very much value-laden process. Reaching consensus on the desired future is one of the most difficult parts of the whole endeavor, yet it is absolutely critical if there is to be any hope of successful implementation of the planning process and any constructive change. The desired future is usually a long-range goal that requires several planning cycles, each with its own interim goals, before it is attained.

The objective for planning and change, as we are using them here, is to improve or to change for the better the quality of life for the people involved. The outcome we seek is very similar to Goulet's definition of development.[5] *Development*, as it is used here, covers the entire gamut of changes in which a social system, with optimal regard for the wishes of individuals and other subsystemic components of that system, moves away from a condition of life that is widely perceived in some way as unsatisfactory toward some life condition regarded as "humanly better." Goulet's approach is holistic in that it takes into account all kinds of changes that a social system, or in our case a community, may wish to make. One must remember that direct changes in one subsystem cannot be made without affecting all of the other subsystems and the whole community as well. Of particular importance is Goulet's concern that changes take into account the wishes of individuals and subsystemic components. Collaboration is the desired process for assessment, planning, change, and evaluation, as we continually reiterate. However, collaboration can only take place among people who participate. In deciding on the community's desired future, consultants must constantly be alert for the interests of those who are to be affected by change but who for whatever reason are not participants in the process. Defining a condition that is perceived as unsatisfactory in many instances is easier than reaching a consensus about what would be "humanly better" and even more so than how to arrive at that happy state. Nonetheless, that is the challenge consultants and community members face as they together strive to arrive at mutually agreed-on goals to bring about the desired future.

Much of what guides people's beliefs concerning better or worse conditions as well as the kinds of changes that are acceptable to alter those perceptions are predicated on people's values. Blum[6] identifies values as the keystone of the process that results in the "impetus for change." The normative approach to decision making involves carefully assessing the present state of affairs and comparing it to some other better or more desirable one. If there are discrepancies between the real and the ideal, values will greatly influence the meanings given to these discrepancies as well as to their relative importance in the larger scheme of things. In the process of collaboration, planning participants must therefore learn about each other's values, even though some of the values that collaborative intersystem or planning group members hold may be much more strongly advocated than practiced.

Not surprisingly, the more pluralistic the planning group is, the more points of view will be presented. Many of these points of view about a desired future will be congruent, others will be conflicting. As Coleman and Nixson[7] point out:

> Self-evidently, there is no universal agreement on what these desired conditions should be; individuals certainly have different preferences regarding life style and relationships with the rest of society; and through their political manifestos nations express different collective (majority and minority) views about the desired state of society—views that change through time.

As is the case with nations, communities and aggregates set forth political manifestos about their desires, particularly in a society as politicized as is the United States. A tremendous challenge in the consensus-building process to arrive at a mutually agreed-on desired future is to be sure that it is indeed a consensus and that the needs and wants of minority groups are included. Collaboration must avoid the tyranny of majority as well as of minority interests by seeking the best ways possible to serve the interests of all groups. Another evidence of the need to view planning as cyclic results from the fact that consensus decisions that are made today may have to be changed in the future as circumstances and interests alter.

Consensus building is an art that takes time and requires a variety of skills to implement. It involves negotiation, compromise, and a variety of the other strategies. Unlike many believe, consensus need not be a win-or-lose situation, that is, some groups or individuals give in and others win or gain to reach an agreement. Consensus building may be the contribution of the consultant as a member of the planning group, but this role may be played equally and effectively by any or all other group members. All participants can contribute their consensus-building skills.

Fisher and Ury[1] propose some very useful and practical guidelines that all planning group members can use in negotiating overall goals and the means to attain them. First they caution that participants in the negotiating process should focus on what they call principled negotiation, which seeks "to decide issues on their merits rather than through a haggling process focused on what each side says it will or won't do."[8] Participants should be urged to avoid taking hard-line positions particularly early in the process. Taking positions tends to lock people into them and to prevent their ability to change. The more positions are clarified and defended, the more committed to or against them people become. Finally, the harder one side tries to convince the other that their position is impossible to change, the more difficult later compromise or change will be.[9]

Principled negotiation involves four major points:[10]

1. Separating people from problems
2. Focusing on interests, not on positions
3. Generating a variety of possibilities before deciding what to do
4. Insisting on objective criteria

Separating people from problems. Participants need to work to learn to view themselves as a group of people working to deal with a problem or to reach a decision that will benefit everyone as much as possible. In this way the pitfall of getting adversary positions can be at least reduced. The climate should be one of all being involved together to serve everyone's interests as well as possible.

Focusing on interests, not on positions. Rather than focusing on various people's or groups' positions, participants need to make an effort to find out what kinds of interests they have that give rise to those positions. For example, basic human needs such as security, a sense of belonging, control over one's own life, or economic well-being are often the underlying interests that lead people to assume hard-line positions. For example, it is possible that most total vociferous opposition by retired people to proposals to change Social Security have much more to do with their fears about their economic security rather than their allegiance to Social Security, per se. If other means to assure economic security for retired people were developed, Social Security changes might become a nonissue with them. Finally, most people involved in collaborative efforts represent constituents' interests as well as their own.

We consultants should assume that participants, including us, have multiple interests.

Generating a variety of possibilities before deciding on what to do. Planning group members must brainstorm to come up with as many alternative approaches as possible. This brainstorming process can be used initially for goal identification and then later to decide on means or actions to attain those goals. Participants should encourage creative thinking on everyone's part in generating options, especially options that can result in mutual gain for all involved. Four major obstacles that get in the way of creative brainstorming should be anticipated and avoided:[11]

1. *Reaching premature judgments* by taking on one or another alternative approach before all of the options the group can think of have been defined and discussed. In the section on change in this chapter, we talk about first- and second-order change. If a planning group is ever to have an opportunity to consider second-order change, they must generate and consider unusual, extraordinary, and even weird alternatives.

2. *Searching for a single answer* when in reality there are many ways or approaches to most problems, all of which need to be at least considered before deciding on the best one or ones.

3. *Assuming that the pie's size is fixed* and so options are limited by external or internal constraints. Often such constraints are not as restricting as one thinks. For example, in planning services, if the resource pie is assumed to be only the actual funding for the program, then the pie's size appears to be fixed. There may be other, nonmonetary or in-kind resources that could be used. In the case studies in Chapter 8, we describe how the Area Agency on Aging (AAA) that wanted the assessment of the elderly aggregate did not give up the idea just because it didn't have the funds. Instead it enlarged the pie by approaching the community health nursing faculty members on Nursing Dynamics Corporation's Board about the possibilities of combining the agency's needs for person power with the faculty member's needs for student field experiences. In this way what originally appeared as a fixed pie, win-or-lose situation was turned into a winning game for all.

4. *Thinking that solving their problem is their problem* is a variation of blaming the victim.[12] Again, if consultants come from a systems perspective, there cannot be "their" problems but only "our" problems that all must work on together. To return to the Social Security change example, people who are less than 65 years of age cannot view Social Security as an older people's problem. Young people, too, will retire some day and, unless retirement economic security issues have been resolved, the problem of economic insecurity will occur for these people as well.

Insisting on objective criteria. Objective criteria or fair standards include market value, precedent, professional standards, scientific judgment, cost, equal treatment, and tradition. Any one or more of these objective criteria can be called on to help evaluate proposed goals or means by more rational criteria than a majority vote or by the sheer power of one interest over others. Fisher and Ury summarize the value of using objective criteria in this way: "By discussing such criteria rather than what the participants are willing or unwilling to do, neither party need give in to the other; both can defer to a fair solution."[13]

Following some of the processes we have suggested here facilitates the planning group's work in collaboratively reaching consensus about goals and means to attain them. Collaboration is not an easy process, nor is it rapid. However, collaboration by those affected helps to ensure that the goals the group selects are adhered to and the means for their attainment are acceptable and therefore are actually followed.

Even when the collaborative process brings agreement on the goal, it is often so globally stated as to defy operation, much less evaluation. For example, the goal for the Apollo space program was very clear. In 1960 President Kennedy promised that the United States would have a man on the moon by 1970. This kind of clear-cut technical goal could be and was translated into action and achievement. The goal for restoring United States cities, proposed by the same president, did not fare nearly as well. The reasons include the goal's vagueness, which prohibited action, as well as the sheer magnitude of the job involved and the number of virtually unmanageable variables.[14,15] Planning group members must not only agree on the plan's goals but also must ensure that the mutually agreed-on goals are stated in behavioral and measurable terms so that the actions they require can not only be taken, but the results can be measured.[16]

Actions and resulting outcomes. Outcomes are the part of planning that derive from implemented actions. Change is usually the outcome. At other times, the participants may make a conscious decision *not* to institute change. In either case, the group implements mutually agreed-on action. We are not laissez faire planners and therefore do not advocate that approach to planning. Thus we are concerned with acting and intervening rather than with being content to let matters take their own course unaided—or hindered. Many planning endeavors never reach the stage of trying to agree on, much less to implement, actions. Some groups seem to derive considerable benefits from endless assessments, or as this activity is also known, planning to plan. Planning to plan also enables planning groups to avoid making either difficult decisions or taking controversial or risky actions. Although a nonaction or planning-to-plan approach may keep the participants busy, it will not bring about planned change nor move the target community or its aggregate closer to the mutually agreed-on goal or desired future.

Evaluation of outcomes and their consequences. This is the final stage of one planning cycle and the initial assessment stage of the next. Viewed in this way, the cyclic nature of planning is more clear. Evaluation of outcomes and their consequences means looking at the immediate and long-term effects of the actions that participants decided to take. If for example the goal is to increase the numbers of young people participating after school in certain kinds of community recreational activities, quantitative outcome evaluation would focus on the actual increase in the number of young people involved in those activities. A qualitative outcome measure would focus on the results of the young people's experiences in the recreational programs, such as enhanced peer support, learning new social and teamwork skills, and increased self-esteem. Assessing the consequences of this outcome involves looking at the changes that participation in such activities may make on indicators such as youth crime rates, loitering, drug abuse, and so forth. Assessment of these kinds of consequences of changes that result from planning actions requires long-term follow-up. This follow-up should be an integral part of the planning evaluation. We discuss a number of evaluation approaches in Chapter 7.

Obviously this definition of planning and our discussion of it are heavily based in systems theory (see Chapter 1). Because communities are made up of interdependent subsystems and are themselves interdependent parts of larger systems, planning groups not only must consider the influencing forces on their planned changes from all these systems but also must recognize that the changes they seek to bring about in any one system or subsystem will affect all of the others. Planning groups must be aware of this rippling effect throughout the planning process.

Guidelines for planning

In most sectors of society, planning goes on in many ways and is conducted by numerous groups. Often there is little or no coordination or communication between groups about their plans. In capitalistic endeavors that are bent on maximizing individual and corporate profits, this may be an effective approach to planning. Our belief is that in fields where public welfare is involved and where public funds are to be spent, coordinated planning efforts are essential. Here we focus our discussion on the health and human services field.

One of the most notable approaches in recent history in the United States toward comprehensive planning has been in the area of planning for health. In 1966 the Congress enacted PL 89-749, the Comprehensive Health Planning Act of 1966. This act and its extension, PL 93-641, The National Health Planning and Resources Development Act of 1974, were landmarks in that they sought to provide coordinated planning efforts to enable communities to control their own health services. Before their enactment there had been all sorts of planning laws for hospital construction, mental health, and other segments. These two laws also mandated consumer participation through the requirement that at least 51% of the members of decision-making groups had to be consumers, that is, persons who did not earn their living in any health or health-related service. To provide for both comprehensive planning possibilities and consumer participation in one statute was a real breakthrough. Early in the 1980s the Reagan Administration saw fit, pursuant to its deregulatory if not

antiregulatory philosophy, to virtually repeal the National Health Planning and Resources Development Act through the budgetary process. Funding for activities
under this law has been so severely curtailed as to make it impossible for activities to
continue in most areas. The people of the United States are therefore now left to
their own state and local devices and to those of various vested interest groups to find
a way to plan for the health needs of communities or aggregates as best they can. In
one sense, the absence of statutory authorities for planning for health may be a
blessing, since it clears the way for local communities or their specific aggregates to
deal with their own needs. On the other hand, it sets up a real climate of competition, where communities or aggregates must strive to get what they can, even if this
is done at the expense of other aggregates or communities. Whatever the pros and
cons, this is the situation we face in the United States in the early 1980s. The case
study in Chapter 7 is an example.

Since human service workers as planning participants are basically free at this
point to pursue health planning, although with little government support or sanction,
we must search for whatever guidelines might be helpful to us in the process. In 1977
the World Health Organization suggested guidelines for planning for health; some of
which we discuss here.[17]

Population-based planning. Planning should be population based. The fundamental question to be addressed here is who is the population with whom consultants
shall plan? Are they the residents of a specific geopolitical area? Are they the members of an aggregate, such as the elderly or parents of retarded persons? Are they
members of a profession or occupation? Are they all people who are subject to some
kind of risk factor, such as radioactive exposure or dangerous levels of certain pol-
lutants? Defining the target population is obviously essential. Human services workers must know who they are and where they are to elicit their participation in the
planning process so that their needs, wants, and priorities, as well as the needed
actions can be accurately assessed. Defining the target population or population base
sounds simple—often deceptively so. Once the target population is defined, subsequent guidelines can be sought.

Epidemiology and social studies. "Epidemiology and social studies are the fundamental health planning sciences, dealing with the behavior of diseases, individuals, and groups."[17] This guideline stresses the need for scientifically gathered, analyzed, and reported data as a baseline for planning for health. Throughout this book
we emphasize the need for comprehensive assessment of the target community
population, aggregate, or group before planning begins. This is a lengthy and expensive process but is essential nonetheless. Chapters 5, 6, 7, and 8 are devoted to
some of the techniques and tools that can be used to study target systems. Statistics
and biostatistics are also essential tools in epidemiology and social studies.

Indicators and proxy measures. "Indicators and proxy measures should be used
for attributes and events that are not easy to measure directly."[17] This is a useful

guideline for assessment and planning. Many of the most important factors to be assessed are the most difficult to define, much less measure. As we discuss in Chapter 6, indicators are often elusive. Great care must be taken to ensure that the indicators and proxy measures used are indeed valid and reliable ones for the phenomena that must be measured, as well as for target systems.

Health. "Health is conceived of as 'the essence of productive life.' All sectors of society affect health."[17] This guideline calls for a comprehensive approach to health that involves all parts of the community. This philosophical approach to health emphasizes that virtually everything affects health and vice versa. There is an increasing recognition throughout the world that a healthy population is a more productive population and so is a great national resource. The planning group needs to bear this fact in mind in defining goals and the means to attain them. The actions that have the greatest impact on health may be in another sector. For example, the infant mortality rate is increasing in some states in the United States where unemployment is very high and so a number of families no longer have the health insurance that was available to them through their employment. Although infant mortality is a frequently used health indicator, its increase in these states is associated with an economic as well as a health situation.

Appropriate services. Services must be appropriate, adequate, and acceptable in the existing circumstances. Many of the goals the planning group will address will be focused on the development or expansion of services for some target aggregate or for the whole community. In this era of shrinking resources for health and related services, we must be sure that services are really needed, that existing services cannot be combined in innovative ways to meet needs, and that innovative ways to combine services that are created are indeed what the people who will use them want. *Appropriate, adequate,* and *acceptable*—all terms that must be operationally defined, preferably by the people who use them—are all important criteria for service development and evaluation. To this list we add affordable, accessible, and available when and where they are needed.

Virtually everyone who writes about planning proposes guidelines, steps, phases, or similar "how tos." Rather than reproduce more of them here, we refer you to a few that you may find useful.[6,18,19,20]

Selected tools for planning

There are many tools available to assist planning groups to reach decisions and to organize their efforts. We present two here that have been particularly useful to us. Decision trees help planning groups to visualize alternatives and their consequences in the process of making decisions. This kind of visualization makes people more aware of the risks or chances that selecting various alternatives involves. Decision trees are particularly valuable tools in contingency planning. Program evaluation review technique (PERT) is both a planning and a control tool. Again, the visualization of the PERT network helps participants to see relationships between activities and to better realize the importance of timing and dependence on the appropriate sequencing of events.

Decision trees. Decision trees are a management tool that is used extensively in making investment, production, and marketing decisions. Decision trees can also be very useful to health and social planning groups in assisting them to weigh alternative courses of actions. The fact that decision trees, as illustrated in Fig. 2, are graphic presentation-making processes makes them very useful in working with groups from varied backgrounds.

Fig. 2 shows the decision tree we used to obtain an adequate sample for our assessment of elderly people's knowledge and use of the services described in Chapter 8. The legend at the lower left shows that the squares on the tree are decision points; the circles are points where chance events occur; and the half diamonds indicate consequences of each of the possible outcomes of the chance events.

The real advantage of a decision tree is that the technique enables participants to visualize different outcomes of decisions and their consequences. It is an effective aid to contingency planning, since all can see what the other alternatives are if one outcome is not forthcoming. Contingency planning is based on "what ifs": What if one alternative does not work? What if we can't obtain the sample we want? Contingency planning seeks to help planning groups anticipate these kinds of questions and to be ready to pursue an alternative course of action. The decision tree helps to make the possible contingencies, alternatives, and consequences clearer through visualization, as in Fig. 2.

In our example, our original plan was to obtain the Social Security lists with the names and addresses of all of the people 65 years of age and over in the county. From these lists we could then draw a systematic random sample of people to contact to invite to participate in the assessment. Had we been able to do that, the decision tree would have been chopped off with only that one branch. Such was not the case, however.

Because of our prior experience with attempts to use the Social Security lists for similar kinds of assessment purposes, we were well aware of the contingency of being forced to consider other approaches for obtaining a sample for the assessment. Thus our decision tree in Fig. 2 begins with an event, not a decision. Our first choice of contingency was to advertise in local public and senior media for volunteers to participate in the assessment. In this way we hoped to obtain access to people who were not already part of the senior services network and so were not already clients of the services we would be assessing. This was an attempt, in the absence of the opportunity to obtain a random sample from the total elderly population in the county, to obtain as unbiased a sample as we could, given that the subjects were volunteers (see Chapter 5).

Advertising involved chance; either we would obtain sufficient volunteers to

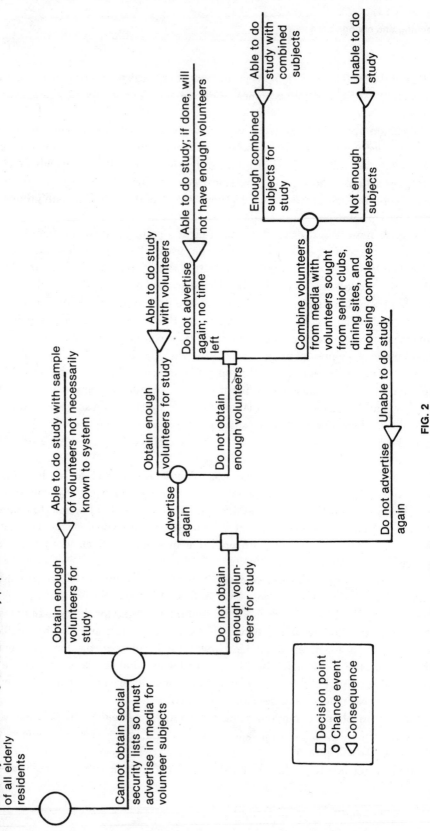

FIG. 2

Decision tree for obtaining elderly persons for assessment of their knowledge and use of senior services.

conduct the assessment or we would not. If we did obtain enough, then obviously we would go ahead with that group of volunteers. If we did not obtain sufficient numbers of volunteers through advertising, we would have to do one of two things: advertise again or forget the whole idea. If we advertised again, there were once again the same two possibilities: we would obtain enough people or we would not. If we obtained enough, we would continue the plan and assess those people. If not enough people responded to the second advertisement, we had to make other decisions.

Anticipating some of the problems we might encounter with persuading people to volunteer for the assessment through our explanations in the media, we had a contingency plan. If all else failed, the final option we could pursue was to ask our colleagues at senior centers, senior clubs, senior dining sites, and senior housing projects for access to their clients or residents so that we could explain the assessment to them in person and invite them to participate. The reason this was a last resort was that virtually all of the elderly people we would obtain through this method would be very much involved in many of the services we were assessing. Although they could give us their valued opinions on the services they knew, they were a much more skewed group of respondents than we had hoped to obtain. The skew, in this case, was very much toward considerable knowledge about and involvement with many of the services, more so than we suspected was true of the total elderly population in the county. Since we did not obtain nearly the number of volunteers from the media advertising that we had hoped for, we were forced to use the last-resort contingency of seeking subjects from within the senior services network. Although the combined group of volunteers from both the media advertisements and the personal contact at senior sites was still quite small, we conducted the assessment. We made very clear to those involved in the survey the limitations that this kind of sampling procedure produced with regard to the generalizability of the results.

As Fig. 2 illustrates, drawing this kind of decision tree on the blackboard or on butcher paper during the discussion of plans and contingencies can be very useful in helping planning group members to see the possibilities and their consequences and to participate in the decisions that result. As the tree illustrates, each branch or possibility is carried out until it can go no further. All of the possible alternatives end in one or another consequence: ability to do the study or inability to do the study. Obviously any of those decision points could be the start of its very own decision tree. The cyclic nature of planning is thus revisited.

Program evaluation review technique (PERT). Once the planning group has made its decisions about what shall be done, tools are needed to implement them. PERT is one of those tools. Developed in the 1950s for use in such projects as the Polaris submarine, PERT has been used in business, health, and social planning as well.[21,22,23] The PERT network is another opportunity to use visualization to help planning group members to see relationships and to appreciate the importance of timing and sequencing.

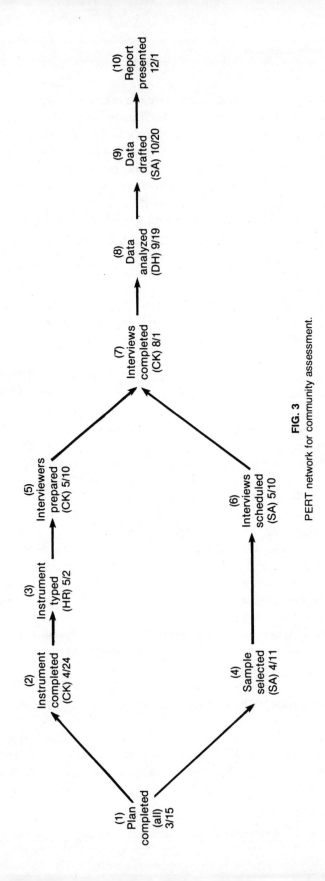

FIG. 3

PERT network for community assessment.

Fig. 3 is an example of a PERT network for carrying out a community assessment using interviews. This is a somewhat more elaborate PERT network than many in that, in addition to listing the actual events (1 through 10), the dates when they are to be completed and the initials of the person who is responsible for seeing that the indicated deadline is met also appear in the network. We like to prepare PERT networks to use as control tools. The final network can be displayed in a place where all involved can see it and so be reminded of times and responsibilities. Copies can also be given to people who are responsible for various events.

The network is prepared by first listing all of the events or completed activities and then ordering them in chronological sequence. Care must be taken here to be sure that no events are omitted. Next, events whose activities can be undertaken simultaneously are identified. In the case of Fig. 3, the selection of the respondents and scheduling of interviews can take place at the same time that the instrument is being finalized, typed, and the interviewers are being prepared. Neither of these sets of events is dependent on the other for its completion. However, both must be finished before the interviewing can actually begin. Once the planning group has identified all of the events that must take place between the completion of the plan and the presentation of the final report, as in this example, the events are numbered sequentially as they will appear on the final network.

The next step is to determine what activities are actually involved in getting from one event to another. Table 2-1 is the list of activities that correspond to the intervals between the events they follow and precede. For example, the activity between

TABLE 2-1

Activities for the PERT network for a community assessment

Event interval	Activity	T_e (in workdays)*	T_e for simultaneous activities
1 to 2	Complete, pretest, and revise assessment instrument	23	
1 to 4	Obtain sample		18
2 to 3	Type and duplicate instrument	6	
4 to 6	Contact respondents and arrange appointments for interviews		17
3 to 5	Train interviewers	6	
5 to 7	Conduct interviews as scheduled	58	
7 to 8	Tabulate and analyze data	35	
8 to 9	Write report	24	
9 to 10	Revise, complete, and type report	28	

*Total calendar workdays needed to complete the project: 180; total person workdays needed to complete the project: 214.

events 1 and 4 is to obtain the sample. As we point out in the decision tree in Fig. 2, this is sometimes not an easy task. The activities that must go on between events 1 and 2 are the completion, pretesting, and revision of the instrument.

The second process regarding the activities is to calculate how long each activity will take to complete. This is a critical step, since these calculations will tell the planning group whether they can make their assigned deadline using usual means. If there isn't enough time, they will have to expend additional resources because standard operating procedures take too long. These time calculations or estimates are listed under the T_e, estimate time, heading in Table 2-1. The formula for estimated time is:

$$T_e = \frac{a + 4m + b}{6}$$

when a = the shortest time possible to complete the activities needed between events. For example, typing the final instrument by using emergency typing facilities and paying extra for them could be accomplished in 2 working days rather than the average of 5.

when m = the average time needed to complete an activity. Again in the case of typing, the average is 5 days for staff to complete a project of that size under normal circumstances.

when b = the longest time it would reasonably take to complete a given activity. For typing the instrument, the estimate might be 15 working days, or three times the average length of time needed.

Thus the T_e for typing the instrument using this example would be calculated:

$$T_e = \frac{2 + 20 + 15}{6}$$

$$T_e = 6+ \text{ working days}$$

The estimated times for all of the activities in this PERT example are calculated in the same way and are displayed as shown in Table 2-1. Note that only one set of times for simultaneously occurring activities is figured when calculating the calendar time needed for a project. However, all T_es for all activities, simultaneous or not, are part of the total person time needed for the project. Thus the person time needed exceeds the calendar time by 35 person workdays.

If the planning group has the luxury of more or less setting its own deadline for completing its work, the PERT network can be set up from event 1 through event 10, using the times indicated by the T_e formula. Using this approach, the project would be due to be finished on the date that the PERT network shows to be the reasonable estimated time to complete it. In reality, at least in the reality of our experience, the planning group almost always has a deadline imposed from outside that it must tailor its projects to meet. For example, if the assessment in the PERT example was being conducted as a needs assessment for a grant proposal, the planning group would have to have the assessment done and reported before the grant proposal was due so that the data could be included in the proposal. When the group is functioning under an imposed deadline, the PERT network can be constructed backward, that is, from the due date back to the present. The same T_e formula is used to calculate how long the project would take under ordinary circumstances. If, in working backward from due date to present date, the group finds that there is not enough time to accomplish the project as calculated, then contingency plans must be made to get it done faster. More interviewers could be hired to speed up the interviewing process; extra staff could be used to prepare instruments and final reports faster. All of these speed-up alternatives are possible; they all cost more money or mean that resources have to be borrowed from other jobs. These additional costs must be calculated into the overall cost of the assessment and weighed against the possible benefits. If the assessment is important enough to complete on time, the extra resources needed will have to be found and paid for. At least with PERT as a planning adjunct, the planning group will know some of the contingencies it is up against and so can plan as realistically as possible to address them.

Advice from one consultant to another

The following is an overview of a number of factors that we have found useful from our experiences as consultants to consider in collaborative planning efforts. They influence not only our own involvement but also community members' participation in the planning process and hence its outcomes.

Consultant's values. These include personal values as well as values acquired through professional educational experiences and associations with professional colleagues. Consultants should also be aware that our values may be influenced by the organizations or agencies in which we are employed. Personal and professional values guide the choices made and the actions taken and are often the basis for differences with the communities with whom consultants work. Therefore, consultants must strive to be aware of our own values and their impact throughout the planning process. As long as collaboration, as described in this chapter, is the overall model for working together and principled negotiation is the means, then all actors are encouraged to share their own thoughts and priorities.[1] This sharing also pertains to consultants in the collaborative process. The overall aim is to work together in a situation in which everyone believes that her or his values are respected in the process of striving to reach outcomes that are of benefit to all.

Community's cultures. The United States is one of the most culturally pluralistic societies in the world. This pluralism is mirrored in the composition of many communities. Race, religion, and linguistic and ethnic backgrounds are included in our operational definition of culture. When consultants plan with the community system as a whole, we must be sure that we do the following:

1. Find out what cultural groups are represented in the community and what their values and beliefs are in general and specifically about the area the planning process will address. This will help consultants to understand many of the interests underlying the positions taken by members of various cultural groups concerning issues.
2. Learn who the influential people are in each cultural group and invite them to participate or to send a representative to be a member of the planning group. Seeking representation raises the dilemma of what representation really is and how it can best be brought about. Can people sent to represent others really do so? If they are sent to represent their constituency's bottom-line position, from which they cannot deviate, negotiation and real collaboration are virtually precluded. If representatives come willing to fully participate in collaborative efforts that result in mutual benefit for all groups, the results may not serve the interests of any one constituency as well as some of its members will want. This dilemma is not unique to collaborative planning efforts but is a potential in all situations where one or a few try to represent many. Consultants should encourage and facilitate as needed representatives remaining in close two-way communication with their respective constituents to enable the constituents to be informed and to provide input and feedback to the planning group through their representatives.

Aggregates may be more culturally homogeneous than are many communities, so consultants may need to be concerned with only one or two diverse points of view rather than many. Nonetheless, consultants should be aware that considerable cultural pluralism may exist even in small aggregates and so should be careful not to overlook potential culturally based influences on planning group members.

Traditions and current practice. There is an old adage that there's no reason for something being done a certain way, except that it is policy. The same kind of attitudes toward traditions and current practices may exist in communities and aggregates with whom consultants work. As with cultural diversity, the most effective way to deal with traditions and current practices is to be aware of them and their influence on the planning endeavor at hand. Evidence of many of the community traditions will emerge in discussions, and current practices often can be identified through observation. Consultants should be particularly alert to the possibility of infringement on traditions and current practices when alternative approaches that are suggested for dealing with a problem meet with immediate rejection by community members in the planning group, even though the alternatives appear perfectly plausible to the consultants. Consultants must do the best we can to help the planning group avoid the pitfall of becoming entrenched in traditions and precedents to the exclusion of different approaches to needs and wants that hold the potential for increased mutual benefit. This will be further explored in the discussion of second-order change.

Community's attitudes toward planning. Attitudes toward planning and planned change may vary greatly among target aggregates and communities with whom consultants may work. Some may want to control the planning process to ensure that *their* desired outcomes result. Examples of such aggregates might include parents of severely mentally retarded or physically handicapped children and the families of very frail elderly. These groups may feel that their needs and concerns will continue to be neglected unless they make concerted efforts to control the process.

At the other extreme, some aggregates and communities may not want any planning at all. Theirs is a laissez faire attitude toward events, allowing whatever happens to occur without interference from them or from others. Planned change is not a value for such groups and we consultants who do value planned change may find that mutually satisfying or beneficial outcomes are not forthcoming from collaboration with these groups. We as consultants may seek to work with other groups who more closely share our preference for planned change.

In between these attitudes of total planning and laissez faire planning are a number of other possible positions with regard to desirability of planned change and how to bring it about. Blum's conceptualizations of these positions can be viewed as a continuum.[24] The consultant should make every effort to learn approximately where on this continuum lie the attitudes of the aggregates or communities toward planning. This information can serve as one guide to the extent of their commitment to change through planning. In this era of uncertainty and rapid technological and social development, change to accommodate, anticipate, or prevent events is a constant. Also the attitudes toward planned change of community members who participate in the planning group may change over time as a result of their experience with collaborative planning.

Congruency of plans with resources. A previously stated caution was that planning groups should not be constrained with the idea that the resources pie is totally fixed, especially when considering possible alternative approaches to a given situation. Nonetheless, consultants must be realistic and consider what resources we can reasonably expect to have to carry out the plans. Until the late 1970s many health and social planning groups functioned with little regard to resource availability, or so it seemed. They felt, with a great deal of public support, that their mandate was to meet needs first and then to worry about resources. This attitude seemed particularly prevalent in medical care where technological explosions and a variety of other factors drove costs and prices for medical care up more rapidly than was the case for most other items on the consumer price index. However, budget priorities, especially in the early 1980s at the federal level, have been altered. Taxpayers are increasingly reticent to pass bond issues to support education, medical, and other human service expansion. Competition for what appears to be fewer tax dollars is growing more vicious as many health and human service programs vie for their very survival. To fail to take resource availability into account, regardless of how pressing an assessment shows the needs of the community to be, is not only courting failure but is also professionally irresponsible and risks raising false hopes. This latter point of raising false hopes is potentially problematic if the target aggregate or community is one that has little experience with change in which the group gained more than it lost.

Use of tools to aid communication. Many community members of planning groups are new to the processes of planned change. Therefore, consultants need to use all of the innovative techniques available to help us to communicate our ideas and to understand what is being done. Clark and others[25] give the example of an urban redevelopment planning program that asked participants to photograph what they liked and did not like in the renewal area so that all could clearly visualize them. Earlier in this chapter there are examples of decision trees and PERT networks, both of which are visual presentations of complex relationships that can be used to aid understanding (see Figs. 2 and 3).

Consultants must bear in mind that many people from communities who participate in the planning group are experts in their own fields or professions, but not necessarily in the subject matter under study. Some may be unfamiliar with many of the components of planning and public life that we consultants take for granted because of our professional socialization. For increasing numbers of citizens, English is a second language. We know from working with the elderly that many of them had only an elementary school education many years ago. Although they are boundless reservoirs of experiential information, many are short on "book learning." Visual acuity and hearing acuity also may be problems for the elderly. This kind of diversity in educational background, experience, and facility with written and spoken English can occur in any of the planning groups in which one participates. Meaningful and effective collaboration cannot occur when any of the community participants are unclear about the issues under discussion. Consultants need to help ensure that participants understand by using every means possible.

Involvement of other agencies. Most geographical areas, particularly urban ones, have a number of health and human services agencies. One or more of these agencies may have interest in and resources for dealing with the issues the planning group is addressing. Just as consultants strive to ensure that members of the community participate in the planning process from the beginning, so we should also discover what agencies or organizations might also be interested and useful and urge their involvement. Many areas have social service councils or other bodies where representatives of agencies with services in a geographical area or for a particular aggregate come together at regular intervals to share information and coordinate their services. In the county where the major part of the assessment activities described in the case study took place (see Chapters 7 and 8), the Agency Council, where representatives of all of the agencies in the community that were concerned with the elderly regularly met, was an invaluable resource for our efforts. We were fortunate that the group was already well established when we did some of our work. A useful spin-off of the planning process could be the beginning of such a social agency coordinating group if one does not already exist in the target community.

Nothing like success. Henrik Blum repeatedly admonishes students to start with a project that has a reasonable chance of success. That admonition is still valid. Many communities and aggregates have had very little positive outcomes from their efforts to make change. Sometimes the resulting frustration boils over into violence, as happened in the 1960s. In more instances people tend to become apathetic and withdraw from public participation, citing the reason, "Nobody cares what I think anyway." These are the very people whose participation is terribly important to the success of any planning activity that affects them. Consultants need to make every effort not only to persuade them to join in collaborative planning but also to ensure that they derive some benefit from their participation per se as well as contributing to the planning group's endeavors.

To be sure, the planned outcome or mutually agreed-on goal of the planning process is the major objective toward which the collaborative planning group works. However, consultants should not become so caught up in this major activity as to lose sight of the need to assist community participants to improve their own organizational skills and to build community competence. Cottrel discusses eight essential conditions to look for in assessing community competence. They are:

1. Commitment to the community as worthy of substantial effort to sustain and enhance it
2. Self-other awareness and clarity of situational definitions
3. Articulateness in expressing views, attitudes, needs, and intentions
4. Communication
5. Conflict containment and accommodation
6. Participation in which members contribute to definitions of goals as well as to ways and means for attaining them
7. Management of relations with the larger society
8. Machinery for facilitating participant interaction and decision making[26]

Goeppinger and her colleagues are working to further apply these essential components so that they can be better used to assess a community's competence.[27] The same criteria and processes can be applied to aggregate assessment. The more competent the community and aggregate become, the more likely that they will be able to function with increasing self-confidence and independence. The most important consequence of collaborative planning and the greatest tribute to consultants is for the community or participants to be able to say at the end that they did it by themselves and that they know how to do it again.

● ● ●

Much of the advice we have discussed here consists of a variety of factors that influence a collaborative planning process. Many are obvious; all are important. Of course there are others that each of you has already experienced or will experience as you work in planning activities with members of target aggregates and communities. You may find it helpful to make a checklist of these and other factors to bear in mind as you work with others in planning for their needs and wants. Such a checklist could well help you to remember these and other important factors that otherwise might be overlooked.

Summary

This discussion of planning has focused on an operational definition of planning that stresses collaborative relationships with the active and continuous involvement of people who will be affected by the changes that planning brings about. We provide examples of two planning tools, decision trees and PERT networks, that not only help to organize, direct, and control planning but are also visual tools and so can help participants to see as well as hear what is being discussed and decided. As with all tools, it is important to remember that no matter how fascinating they are to develop and play with, they are means to other ends.

CHANGE

The remainder of this chapter deals with change. The authors focus on change as the outcome of the planning process and so feel that a quick review of some of the most salient aspects of change theory in this context is appropriate. As an orientation to the types of change, we discuss rational-empirical, normative-reeducative, and power-coercive types. We follow this with a presentation of first- and second-order change and their implications for much of what health and human service professionals try to do. We conclude with some ideas about applying change strategies in situations where ambiguity and uncertainty are rife.

Types of change strategies

Chin and Benne[28] describe three types or groups of change strategies, all of which have relevance to community and aggregate assessment.

Rational-empirical change. The basic assumption for rational-empirical change strategies is that people are able and willing to make decisions on the basis of the facts or empirical information presented to them, particularly if this evidence indicates that they will derive some benefit from the change. For example, people will often be skeptical about the value of community assessment activities that involve gathering information from them. Very often they will reconsider this attitude and agree to participate if they receive information that there may be direct benefits to them from their participation, such as the development of programs or services that could be of value to them and those close to them. When we were doing the needs assessment for a grant proposal to develop an adult day-care program, we were quick to point out to both individual and agency respondents what the program might do for them if it were developed. In short, the rational-empirical approach to change involves giving people answers to the very basic question, "What's in this for me?" This question is not a selfish one, but rather a very realistic one that needs to be answered very clearly before one can expect community participation, much less change.

Normative-reeducative change. This approach to change is predicated on the belief that people have values, norms, and attitudes that influence, if not direct, their behavior. Their willingness to change, therefore, hinges on their openness to re-examine and possibly alter these values, norms, and attitudes. Giving people the facts alone is not seen as sufficient in this approach to change. In normative-reeducative strategies, efforts are focused on helping people to reexamine their values in the hope that they will come to view situations differently. For example, many of the consumers and health care providers we worked with in comprehensive health planning and health systems agencies originally came to the planning group with very negative attitudes toward the whole business. They seemed to feel that these planning groups and their efforts were just another meaningless gesture by government and powerful health care providers. In the course of working in collaboration with other members of these planning groups, some of their attitudes changed. As these alterations in attitudes occurred, so did consumers' commitments to the kinds of things these planning groups were trying to accomplish. They became open to looking at information in a very different way and to asking questions about how that information could be used. Until their attitudes and values toward the planning process and their roles in it changed, there was little cooperation and less progress. Where their basic distrust was not at least lessened, planning groups, particularly those that strove for collaborative involvement, were stymied. The point here is that those who are involved in planned change must be aware of the values and attitudes others bring to these processes. Change efforts through normative reeducation may have to begin here. If unsuccessful, those efforts will probably get no further.

Power-coercive change. The third type of change strategies generally involves political or economic sanctions or applications of power. For Alinksy[29] and community organizers of his ilk, power-coercive strategies are the strategies of choice from the outset. For others these strategies are a last resort. If rational-empirical and normative-reeducative change strategies fail, force, albeit legitimate, is often tried (see Chapter 3). An example of a power-coercive change strategy that has failed, in our opinion, is busing to achieve racial integration in schools. Although the force of law has been clearly behind busing, the law has been subverted in many places because people apparently see too little rational-empirical evidence of sufficient benefit for them to comply. Perhaps even more detrimental to achievement of the desired outcome of this approach to integration is that it was not preceded by effective efforts to change public values and attitudes toward integration. In short, effective normative-reeducative change was not brought about first. This example epitomizes the weaknesses of the use of power-coercive change strategies unless and until public attitudes and desires have changed to support the laws or other sanctions. Again there is the old saying that the most effective laws are those that legitimate common practice rather than initiate it.

Power-coercive change strategies virtually negate collaborative planning and change efforts. For this and the reason already given for the shortcomings of power-coercive strategies, we strongly recommend that they be avoided unless all else literally fails. For those of you who want to explore the concept of power further, there are many sources you can consult.[30-36]

First- and second-order change

"The more things change, the more they are the same" is a French proverb that may not appear at first to make sense. Its meaning will become more clear as we discuss first- and second-order change. Watzlawick and others[37] use the theory of groups and the theory of logical types from the field of general mathematical logic for the development of the concepts of first- and second-order change. We draw much of the basis for our discussion of these concepts from their work, as others have done.[38]

First-order change. First-order change is most common. It is change that is brought about in a system without the system itself being changed. The basic rules are not changed, nor is the system's structure altered. The assistance given clients under the heading of "helping them to work the system," is first-order change. Despite the best intentions, all one is really doing is helping clients to make the best they can of a less than desirable situation. They, not the system, adjust and conform. For example, many elderly people believe that they get the "run around" from the staff in the Social Security and Medicare office when they go in to ask about their benefits or their bills. They can't understand the written materials given to them because the language is "legalese," or they may not be able to read it at all because the print is too small, and often the staff are too busy to really sit down and hear their questions before giving them pat answers. All who work with the elderly have heard these tales many times. Actions, however, generally center around helping elderly clients by translating the "legalese" into plain English, getting spectacles for them so they can at least see what is written, and even contacting a colleague in the Medicare office and asking that she or he see the client personally and help.

Now all of this activity is very useful to be sure. Our clients believe that they are being helped, as indeed they are. Consultants feel rewarded because once again we have assisted the people whom the system is supposed to serve to breach the walls of bureaucracy and get what they are entitled to. Everyone has a good feeling of accomplishment—until the next time. Absolutely nothing has really changed and so the same problems will recur to these very clients and to legions of others. If one relies on first-order change, the more things change, the more they remain the same.

Another approach to first-order change is to apply the formula that says "if a little doesn't work, try a lot more of the same thing." This is a particularly popular approach for individuals, aggregates, organizations, and communities that are tradition and precedent bound. Applying more of the same solutions because they have always been used that way and have worked before can lock planning and change efforts into an endless circle of applying band-aids without ever looking for other alternatives. Again everyone is very busy, often to the burnout point, without making any real change that will prevent the recurrence of the same kinds of problems over and over.

There is another approach to all of this—second-order change.

Second-order change. Second-order change focuses on the system, not the system's clients, as the point of change. Second-order change seeks new ways to do things: new approaches and innovative structures and ideas. As we noted in our discussion of planning, some of the reasons planning groups never even consider second-order change are that they jump to premature decisions before considering all of the possible alternatives—particularly the unique or weird ones—and they let tradition stand in the way of innovation even if they come up with innovations.

Second-order change requires new unconventional thinking about problems and needs. A useful group approach might be to come up with all of the usual ways of dealing with problems, the vast majority of which are first-order change approaches, and then to throw the list away and start over from scratch. Now only unusual, off-the-wall kinds of ideas can be brought before the group. The outcome of this kind of brainstorming can be really exciting—and useful. However, before people can get to the point of even thinking about possible second-order change approaches, they have to be helped to move beyond their conventional first-order, tradition-bound approach to change.

A well-known puzzle will help to clarify a basic principle of second-order change; namely that to make second-order change, one must go outside of the system itself to find a solution.[39] The objective of solving the puzzle is to connect the following nine dots with four straight lines made without lifting the pencil from the paper. Try it.

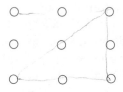

Within the box formed by the boundary of the dots, you are literally boxed into the system by the first-order change logic and will never succeed. The only way to solve the puzzle and connect the dots as directed is to go outside of the system's boundaries as shown.

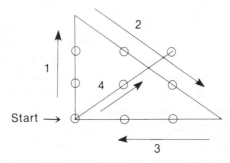

To return to the example with Social Security and Medicare, a second-order change perspective means that one would have to look at what is wrong with or less than desirable about the system. The objective then would become to fix the system to meet client needs rather than the first-order change approach used for fixing the clients to conform to the system. It is probable that endless findings from evaluations of public and private health and human services systems clearly indicate the need for changes in the systems themselves. They are not adequately addressed, if they are addressed at all, because most human service workers cannot deal with change of the magnitude required to really make a change. As Watzlawick and others point out:

> It is our experience that second order change appears unpredictable, abrupt, illogical, etc., only in terms of first order change, that is from within the system. Indeed, this must be so, because, as we have seen, second order change is introduced into the system from outside and therefore is not something familiar or something understandable in terms of the vicissitudes of first order change. Hence its puzzling, seemingly capricious nature. But seen from outside the system, it merely amounts to a change of the premises . . . governing the system *as a whole*.[40]

If assessments and the plans for change that result from them are to have any more than first-order change results, planning groups must learn to seek out and implement second-order changes. To be sure, second-order change involves risks, risks to traditions and to the vested interests of people, aggregates, and communities. Suggestions for second-order change may even jeopardize the consultants' own jobs, but to do less in the face of overwhelming evidence that second-order change is indeed what is required, is to continue to engage in fruitless first-order change activities. Consultants must do something more potentially effective with our skills and energies than to continue what amounts to "rearranging the chairs on the deck of the Titanic in hopes that we will save the ship."

Change: unfinished business

Many who work in social change and health education have long used Lewin's classic three-phase model of planned change: unfreeze, change, and refreeze.[41] They have used this change model whether they chose to employ rational-empirical, normative-reeducative, or power-coercive strategies. To unfreeze, the consultant, change agent, or health educator must first help those with whom she or he works to become ready or, preferably, to actively seek change. Assessment and evaluation data and feedback from the environment can aid people to collaboratively reach the decision that change is needed as well as what kind of change to implement. Groups and individuals who are quite satisfied with the status quo do not want change and so are resistant to unfreezing efforts. They will need what Alinksy[29] refers to as disorganizing efforts to stimulate dissatisfaction with the status quo.

After implementation of the mutually agreed-on change, whatever it is, comes refreezing or stabilization.[42] Refreezing aims at creating a new status quo, albeit different from previous ones. Certainly some pause is needed to enable the planning group to evaluate the instituted changes. However, in this era of uncertainty, ambiguity, and rapid social change, one must be cautious about refreezing too solidly, since needs for subsequent changes are virtually inevitable.

Minkler[43] describes three alternative change approaches:
1. Noncontingent or reformist change
2. Contingent or tentative change
3. Unfinished or changing change

Noncontingent or reformist change. Noncontingent change is based on the classic lewinian model just described.[42] Much of the change involved is first-order change with stability as a desired consequence. Again, when the need for subsequent change arises, this refreezing is a deterrent. In situations where variables are known and the outcomes and consequences of change can be predicted or at least are thought to be predictable, perhaps this approach is warranted. An example of appropriate use of noncontingent change is working with communities to develop antismoking programs, including public education, increased taxation on tobacco products, and laws to restrict smoking in public buildings and restaurants. Since the association of tobacco use and many of our chronic illnesses and leading causes of death is clear, one is on safe ground in using noncontingent or reformist approaches to influence changes in smoking behaviors. Such certainty is a rare commodity.

Contingent or tentative change. Contingent change is based on feedback from the environment and from the consequences of previous changes. In short, it is empirically based and so is subject to change as the empirical data change. This approach enables the planning group to be flexible in response to new information. Although most of the changes involved are of a first order, the system is held in a relatively fluid state and so can adapt more readily to changes in its environment. An example of this kind of change is instituting a pilot program to see how it works before introducing a new service throughout a community. If feedback indicates that the program is workable, it may be both generalized and institutionalized.

Unfinished or changing change. Unfinished change views change as a continuous process rather than as a permanent one. It recognizes that in an age such as this, one must constantly be changing, adapting, and cybernating if one is to survive, much less thrive. In this approach, change is viewed as a constant. A further advantage, as Minkler points out, is that the unfinished approach to change can facilitate movement beyond mere reform, which is first-order change, to system, or second-order change. The focus here is on the process of change more than on its outcomes or products.[44]

Helping those with whom one works to tolerate if not appreciate unfinished change is analogous to Fisher and Ury's warning to avoid premature judgments, seeking single answers and allowing oneself to become locked into specific positions.[1] All of these actions make responses to subsequent indications for change more difficult than they need be. The uncertainty and rapid social change make contingency planning essential so that one can adapt or change the systems in response to altered needs or demands in the environment.

An example that is close to many human service workers is the changes forced by the federal budgets in the early 1980s in many health and human service systems. Reduced funding in general and substantial alterations in federal spending priorities, coupled with taxpayers' apparent aversion to tax increases, have resulted in many agencies having to implement second-order changes to survive at all. Should government priorities and practices continue as they are, even more changes in health and human services systems will be required. Should government policies be substantially altered as a result of upcoming elections, then other changes, perhaps more than most service systems and communities would like, may be forthcoming. Truly change is an unfinished business and must be treated as such.

SUMMARY

Our discussion of planning here has stressed that it is a collaborative, orderly, and cyclic process to attain goals that will move communities and aggregates toward a mutually agreed-on desired future. Collaboration by all groups throughout the process is a keystone. We view change as desirable, inevitable, ubiquitous, and continuous. Both first- and second-order change must be considered and implemented as needed, as communities, organizations, aggregates, and other systems seek input and feedback to enable them to adapt to social and environmental changes. To be frozen is to risk becoming obsolete.

REFERENCES

1. Fisher, R., and Ury, W.: Getting to yes: negotiating without giving in, Boston, 1981, Houghton-Mifflin Co.
2. Arnold, M.F.: Evaluation: a feedback model. In Blum, H.L., editor: Health planning, Berkeley, 1969, University of California, School of Public Health, p. 13.
3. Blum, H.L.: Does planning work anywhere? American Journal of Health Planning 3(3):34-47, 1978.
4. Archer, S.E.: Selected community health process. In Archer, S.E., and Fleshman, R.P., editors: Community health nursing: patterns and practice, ed. 2, North Scituate, Mass., 1979, Duxbury Press, p. 85.

5. Goulet, D.: The cruel choice: a new concept in the theory of development, New York, 1973, Atheneum Publishers, p. 333.
6. Blum, H.L.: Planning for health, ed. 2, New York, 1981, Human Science Press, p. 46.
7. Colman, D., and Nixson, F.: Economics and change in less developed countries, Oxford, 1978, Philip Allan Publishers, Ltd., p. 2.
8. Fisher and Ury, p. xii.
9. Fisher and Ury, p. 5.
10. Fisher and Ury, pp. 11, 17-98.
11. Fisher and Ury, pp. 59-61.
12. Ryan, W.: Blaming the victim, New York, 1971, Pantheon Books.
13. Fisher and Ury, p. 12.
14. Catanese, A.J.: Planners and local politicians: impossible dreams, Beverly Hills, Calif., 1974, Sage Publications, Inc., pp. 56-60.
15. Moynihan, D.P.: Maximum feasible misunderstanding: community action in the war on poverty, New York, 1969, The Free Press.
16. Mager, R.F.: Preparing instructional objectives, Palo Alto, Calif., 1967, Fearon Publishers, Inc.
17. World Health Organization: International collaborative study of medical care utilization, health services: concepts and information for national planning and management, Geneva, 1977, World Health Organization, pp. 108-114.
18. Dever, G.E.A.: Community health analysis: a holistic approach, Germantown, Md., 1980, Aspen Systems Corp.
19. Archer, pp. 69-86.
20. Hyman, H.H.: Health planning: a systematic approach, ed. 2, Rockville, Md., 1981, Aspen Systems Corp.
21. Levine, R.I., and Kirkpatrick, C.A.: Planning and control with PERT/CPM, New York, 1966, McGraw-Hill, Inc.
22. Arnold, M.F., editor: Health programs implementation through PERT: administrative and educational uses, San Francisco, 1966, Western Regional Office, American Public Health Association.
23. Archer, S.E.: PERT: a tool for nurse-administrators, Journal of Nursing Administration 4:26-32, September-October, 1974.
24. Blum, 1978, pp. 56-85.
25. Clark, F.F., Robinson, G.W., and Krauss, R.I.: Getting people involved: experience and techniques in participatory planning, International Development Journal 20:28-31, 1978.
26. Cottrell, L.S., Jr.: The competent community. In Kaplan, B.H., Wilson, R.N., and Leighton, A.H., editors: Further elaborations in social psychiatry, New York, 1976, Basic Books Inc., Publishers, pp. 198-205.
27. Goeppinger, J., and others: Community health is community competence, Nursing Outlook 30:464-467, 1982.
28. Chin, R., and Benne, K.D.: General strategies for effecting changes in human systems. In Bennis, W. and others, editors: The planning of change, ed. 3, New York, 1976, Holt, Rinehart & Winston, Inc. pp. 22-45.
29. Alinsky, S.: Rules for radicals: a pragmatic primer for realistic radicals, New York, 1971, Vintage Books.
30. Archer, S.E.: Selected concepts fundamental to nurses' political activism. In Archer, S.E., and Goehner, P.A., editors: Nurses: a political force, Monterey, Calif., 1982, Wadsworth Health Sciences Division, pp. 71-80.

31. Ashley, J.A.: Hospitals, paternalism, and the role of the nurse, New York, 1976, Teachers' College Press.
32. Bacharach, S.B., and Lawler, E.J.: Power and politics in organizations, San Francisco, 1980, Jossey-Bass, Inc., Publishers.
33. Hawley, W.D., and Wert, F.M.: The search for community power, ed. 2, Englewood Cliffs, N.J., 1974, Prentice-Hall, Inc.
34. Hersey, P., and Blanchard, K.H.: Management of organizational behavior: utilizing human resources, ed. 3, Englewood Cliffs, N.J., 1977, Prentice-Hall, Inc.
35. Kahn, S.: How people get power: organizing oppressed communities for action, San Francisco, 1970, McGraw-Hill, Inc.
36. Shiflett, N., and McFarland, D.E.: Power and the nurse-administrator, Journal of Nursing Administration 8:19-23, March, 1978.
37. Watzlawick, P., Weakland, J.A., and Fisch, R.: Change: principles of problem formation and problem resolution, New York, 1974, W.W. Norton & Co., Inc., Publishers.
38. Donnelly, G.F., Mengel, A., and Sutterley, D.C.: The nursing system: issues, ethics, and politics, New York, 1980, Wiley Medical Publications, pp. 116-123.
39. Watzlawick and others, pp. 24-27.
40. Watzlawick and others, p. 24.
41. Lewin, K.: Group decision and social change, In Maccoby, E., and others, editors: Readings in social psychology, ed. 3, New York, 1958, Henry Holt and Co., Inc., pp. 197-211.
42. Lippett, R., and others: The dynamics of planned change, New York, 1958, Harcourt, Brace & Co.
43. Minkler, M.: Unfreezing Lewin: the case for alternative change strategies in health education, International Quarterly of Community Health Education 1:174-177, 1980-1981.
44. Minkler, p. 175.

3

COMMUNITY ORGANIZATION

Community organization and community development are familiar to many community workers, particularly those in social work and health education. Though others do this type of work on a regular basis, some of us, especially in nursing and education, do not identify our activities as community organizing. Community organization activities are or should be integral in health and social services professions. This chapter presents a number of community organization theories and processes and provides the reader with an example of their application to collaborative planning for change. The authors cannot hope to cover the topic thoroughly in a single chapter; however, we do highlight what we believe are the most significant theorists in the field and demonstrate how community organization, planning, and evaluation are related.

HISTORICAL AND THEORETICAL BACKGROUND

The last 20 years have shown an extensive movement toward communities making decisions for themselves.[1-8] The civil rights movement, the move to community-based programs, local initiatives, and the new federalism have resulted in people from all walks of life becoming intimately involved in programs, such as model cities and health planning, that directly affect their communities. Mandated federal programs provided an opportunity for lay people to participate in community decision making. By designating a number of consumer positions that must be filled on both advisory and policy boards, grass-roots input has been increased. From the city level to the federal level, these boards have helped determine needs and services throughout the nation.

Individual grass-roots participation has been accompanied by the evolution of voluntary and/or professional community organization associations. This involves community groups who join together to instigate a social change such as building affordable housing, demanding better schools, or developing different types of health care services. Spergel[9] describes *community organization,* as used by social scien-

51

tists, as "the natural way or process by which institutions, organizations, and roles of people in a community are interrelated, developed, and changed." He continues to say that the process may focus on people or organizations and may vary from a local functional concern to a massive social movement. Ross[10] defines community organization more comprehensively:

> Community organization . . . has been defined as the process of bringing about and maintaining a progressively more effective adjustment between social welfare needs within a geographic area or functional field. Its goals are consistent with all social work goals in that its primary focus is upon needs of people and provision of means of meeting these needs in a manner consistent with the precepts of democratic living.

What Ross says here about social work is equally applicable to all health and human service activities. Both definitions identify specific components of community organization. The first, process, is a planned movement to achieve a specified outcome. Second, there is the expectation of change. The third area, the democratic precept, identifies community organization as a collaborative process for bringing about change. According to Spergel, community organization became well established by 1874 with the Charity Organization Movement that developed in the United States. This movement involved the wealthy of the community working to help the poor. There was a prestigious aura to the volunteer who devoted time to these causes, and those with money influenced the way society changed. Spergel defines three classes of services prevalent at this time: case work, group work, and community organization.[9] Case work, as the name implies, focuses on problem-solving processes with individual or family clients. Group work extends this process to groups of clients. We have already defined community organization.

Spergel divides the development of community organization into three distinct periods:[9]

1874 to 1917—The movement to strengthen social interventions, such as inter-agency agreements and case conferences

1917 to 1935—The rise of welfare councils and agency federations

1935 to present—The rise of community organization as a practice area of many professions; also a period of theory development

For example, not until 1934 did the concept of self-help and neighborhood involvement become significant. The Chicago Area Project directed its efforts toward dealing with juvenile delinquency in the slums. Project collaborators included the state of Illinois and local community committees. The Chicago Area Project has been used as a model for other low-income neighborhoods. It provides an example of community development from financial and technical dependence on the state to a self-reliant financially independent community organization.

Alinsky used this project as a model for developing his concept of community control.[8] He justified local control by communities as an operationalization of democracy. He saw the alternative to a democratic society as a rule by the elite either in the form of a dictator or by a political aristocracy. He was able to teach communities how to use power to make changes for their benefit. He believed that moral decisions determine human action, despite the corrupting political and social arena in which society finds itself. Words such as compromise have no place in Alinsky's ideology. Poor citizens have the right to organize and to fight for a recognized and effective voice in society. Civil disobedience plays an enormous part in gaining control of power. Alinsky emphasizes educating the organizer in what he calls the ideal elements: "Curiosity, irreverence, imagination, a sense of humor, a bit of a blurred vision of a better world, an organized personality, a well-integrated political ego, and a free and open mind and political relativity."[11]

The community organizer whom Alinsky molds must believe that the end justifies any means and must be willing to put aside the idea that political and social establishments are sacred and inviolate. His is an idealistic, revolutionary stance, a stance that makes followers willing to fight long and hard to bring about desired change.

Ross's goals are very similar to Alinsky's, but his methods are evolutionary rather than revolutionary.[10] Ross believes in working within established social and political systems in collaboration with the people who have power to affect change. Both emphasize citizens' rights to participate in a democratic society. Their methods for this participation are different but not mutually exclusive. The major difference lies in Ross's acceptance that the system exists and can be worked with, whereas Alinsky believes that a reformation must take place through revolution if all else fails. The authors do not subscribe totally to either of these models. We recognize that first-order change,[12] such as Ross advocates, may be appropriate in some circumstances. In others, these evolutionary methods may not be effective, and the kinds of second-order changes that Alinsky advocates are the only way to bring about the desired future that people have defined.

Models of community organization

Ross categorizes his model into three separate components, none of which is mutually exclusive of the others.[13]

Community development. Community development involves efforts to provide for the community's advancement toward changes that are desired. He identifies three types of approaches in community development.

External agency approach. The external agency approach is the basis for agency projects such as VISTA or the Peace Corps, in which individuals are assigned by a sponsoring technically advanced government to help improve living conditions for either American or foreign citizens. More often than not, the programs are initiated by the government structure rather than by the people themselves.

In this category, the community worker works as a technical expert or part of a team that provides expertise to a community to solve a particular problem. This external agent is responsible for assessing and diagnosing the problem and then providing the expertise for the community to deal with it. This goal-directed project has certain expected results for which the external agent is responsible.

Based on his experience and study of Peace Corps volunteers, Rhoades[14] attributed a great deal of volunteer frustation, the indifference of host country nationals to volunteer activity, and the failure of programs to work to "the lack of proper fit between the American model of planned change and the realities of the development situation." He suggests that development agencies should spend more time rethinking their ethnocentric development philosophy and perhaps helping potential volunteers become aware of and clarify their own philosophy and values (see Chapter 4).

We do not advocate the use of the expert external role except in very limited situations where there is no time for or no commitment on the part of the target community or aggregate system to develop a collaborative relationship. Efforts that are tantamount to making changes for people often have negative consequences for the people involved as well as for the programs or other kinds of changes that are instigated.

Multiple approach. The multiple approach involves teams of experts who, as a result of technological changes in a community, provide a variety of services to help the community adjust to them. Often the team identifies and recommends solutions to the community's problem without the involvement of community members in the decision making. Careful thought has to be given to implementing decisions the community had no part in making. More often than not, the results of this multiple approach are useless if not detrimental, as are similar efforts by an individual external expert.

Inner resources approach. The inner resources approach encourages members of the community to do the assessment and diagnosis of the problem themselves. A vested interest in the outcome of planning is likely to develop if the community is involved in the change process from the beginning. Cooperation and mutual goal setting are the major components of this method. This is the one of Ross's three approaches that is at all congruent with the collaborative intersystem model in Chapter 1 (see Fig. 1, p. 16).

Community organization. Community organization refers to "community action and planning."[15] Ross again defines three different approaches, all of which overlap.

Specific content objective approach. The specific content objective approach focuses on a particular problem. Organizations, groups, or agencies use a variety of means to eliminate the problem. This approach can be illustrated by the possible methods for changing a city ordinance involving land use. The process may be a simple and uncomplicated one in which a committee formulates the ordinance, presents it to the planning commission, obtains passage, and receives applause for a job well done. The same desired outcome may become very complicated, depending on the amount of interest and emotion that the issue generates. Representation on the committee may prove to be a complicated stumbling block as various members vie to protect their vested interests. The community itself may be divided on the committee's recommendations, resulting in the need for a series of public hearings so that all groups and individuals can voice their ideas and hear those of others. In the end, because of particular circumstances at a given time in a specific community, the end result may be very different than was originally expected.

General content objective approach. The general content objective approach focuses on the development of a collaborative and coordinated system that allows the representatives of groups to work cohesively toward a specific area of interest. A mental health advisory board, which works to plan, coordinate, and advocate for mental health programs is an example of this approach. This is an ongoing process with continued development of an area being sought as opposed to the pursuit of a single goal.

Process objective approach. The process objective approach uses a network concept in which communication and collaboration between community groups provide opportunities to share responsibility and to initiate action. The focus is on the process, not on the outcome. For example, the community may decide that they wish to join together as a council of agencies to share problems and functions and together seek solutions as a community facing common problems.

Community relations. Community relations are a vital part of community organization. People who have been involved in developing and administering a community group or agency are aware of the importance that relating to community media and other publicity sources has in success or failure of the organization. Ross describes three kinds of community relations strategies.[16] *Public relations* involves the ways an agency projects its image in the community. *Community service* is a method used by an agency to improve its credibility in the community. Business and service clubs may do this by making facilities available for use by other community groups, by buying baseball uniforms for Little League teams, or by providing transportation for the elderly. The benefits derived are twofold: some of the community's needs are served and the business or service club becomes a more accepted part of community life. *Community participation* involves representation from businesses and agencies on committees or task forces that serve the community. For example, members of the Commission on Aging along with representatives from consumer groups, senior services, the real estate bureau, and the city council may meet to consider housing for the frail elderly. Obviously, public relations are enhanced by providing community service and by participating in community planning groups. The agency or group that ignores the community relations component of community work may suffer both a lack of acceptance and a paucity of financial support, since much of the success and support of an agency or business depends on the community's perceptions of its involvement with and commitment to the community.

Rothman describes three models of community organization practice.[17]

Model A: locality development. Locality development focuses on the community's capacity for self-help and thus implies that the community has inner resources to meet many of its own needs. Consensus is the decision-making approach and group discussions are the vehicle for reaching consensus. It assumes that the community is fairly stable and depends on widespread citizen participation in collaboration with members of the power structure for problem solving and decision making. Since this model focuses on a locality, it has application to communities as we have defined them, that is, geopolitical units. Certainly commitment to collaborative planning for community change is based on the belief that communities have the capacity to define and to address their own needs.

Model B: social planning. Social planning is a task-centered, problem-solving approach to addressing a community's substantive problems and needs. The power structure is viewed in this model as the employer and sponsor of activities with less citizen and consumer participation than is the case in the locality development model. Social planning very nearly epitomizes the process that many federally mandated planning and development programs, such as health planning, community mental health, city planning departments, and the like, have followed. Change in this model is largely a result of rational-empirical and normative-reeducative strategies[18] (see Chapter 2).

Model C: social action. Social action is based on shifting power relationships and on institutional change. Clearly this model seeks second-order change.[19] It assumes that segments of the population, who are referred to as victims, are oppressed and will rise up against the power structure that is seen as the oppressor. Change is brought about through actions of mass organizations and political processes. Confrontation, conflict, and direct-action strategies are favored. The critical consciousness-raising work of Freire[20-21] provides additional strategies to help oppressed groups become aware of and actualize their own potential to effect transformation in their society.

Summary

Ross's community development, community organization, and community relations conceptualizations are quite similar to Rothman's locality development and social planning. For comparisons of social-action models, one must look to Alinsky.[8] The model of a collaborative intersystem that combines parts of the consultant- or change-agency system and the target aggregate and community system into a third system assumes both more participation and more innate abilities to identify and deal with needs within aggregates and communities than do any of the other models or approaches we have discussed.

COMMUNITY ORGANIZER ROLES

Ross defines four roles that he believes community organizers play.[23] The *guide* assists communities to attain their goals. The *enabler* is a facilitator who also acts as a catalyst and encourages the community to define common goals and to develop a cooperative atmosphere. The *expert* is a technocrat who provides data analysis and other technical assistance. This role also includes that of a resource person. The *social therapist* assumes a therapeutic stance in helping communities to diagnose and treat their problems. As is the case with most other approaches to role typologies, there are great overlaps and parallels in how various roles are defined. We will therefore confine our discussion to Ross's four general roles, which subsume most others.

Community organizer skills

The skills of the community organizer are derived from several writers.[8,23-25] They include:
1. A working knowledge of community organization theory and process
2. Good planning and assessment skills
3. Knowledge of the community in which organization is taking place
4. Awareness of the power structure and the transfer of power in the community
5. Credibility within the community
6. Dedication to an idea or goal
7. Trust in others and in their abilities
8. The ability to share responsibility
9. Good communication skills
10. Leadership qualities
11. Belief in the democratic process
12. Flexibility to be able to react to the situation and respond appropriately
13. Time-management skills to realistically obtain objectives in reasonable time, acknowledging the constraints and resources available
14. Acceptance that the community, not the individual, is the client
15. Research skills
16. A sense of humor
17. Patience

It may seem that a community organizer must be all things to all people while dressed in a cloak of honesty, goodness, and patience. This is not so. The community organizer can be any one of us. One needs to recognize the strengths one has and be aware of faults and weaknesses as well. This chapter does not suppose that you will become a professional community organizer. What it does aim for is the provision of a theoretical and a structural approach on which the health and human services workers can build in the community process. All of us bring our own biases to the situation. What we must be aware of is that we do not force these biases on others.

CASE STUDY

The problem of a shortage of adequate quality nursing home beds is common to many communities. It is a national problem, one that may become a national emergency, given the increase in the number of elderly projected for the future. In a small city in northern California, that emergency situation has already occurred. The population growth over the past 10 years in the county was 7% while the percentage of elderly increased more than five times that, or 38%. The nursing home beds totalled approximately 1250 a year (already 25% short of the estimated 1500 beds needed in a community of that size). During 1982 almost 200 of these beds had been closed. The events surrounding the closure of some of those 200 beds provide an excellent study in community organization.

Carole Kelly is a community nurse who is involved in this case. She has lived in the county for the past 15 years and has been both a volunteer and a professional health care provider during that period. At the time the nursing home closed, she was serving as a commissioner on the County Commission on Aging. The Commission is an advisory board to the Area Agency on Aging (AAA). Its duties include planning, coordinating, evaluating, and being advocates for programs for the elderly. She was appointed to the Commission as a representative of the city in which the nursing home was closing.

When one lives in a small city, news is often delivered by strange messengers. The first news of the nursing home closure was carried by the children. The local parish priest who worked with the patients at the nursing home and served Mass there frequently was an apparent source. The children themselves often entertained at the nursing home. Other churches and advocate groups, such as the ombudsman program and Love Is the Answer (LITA), also had activities in the nursing home. The nursing home provided an opportunity for the elderly to be involved in community activities. Plans by the nursing home's owners were to replace it with a chemical dependency recovery hospital.

The community felt anger and frustration regarding the closure—anger because it removed the patients from their community and closed a much-needed facility and frustration because someone outside of the city had made the decision about the type of services the city needed.

Attention will be focused, for the moment, at those who ran the nursing home. The managing organization is a subsidiary of a huge, national proprietary organization that provides a variety of health care services in the country. The building itself is owned by a family in a nearby city. They lease the facility to the managing organization. The point we stress here is *proprietary*. The reason stated for the closure was the financial loss that the nursing home had incurred in the previous 2 years. Funding is always a problem for most community services, and no one argues that reimbursement is ever adequate. When stockholders must receive a dividend, the pressure to operate in the black is highly intense. There always has been the question of the compatibility of quality care and profit in nursing homes.[26] It is difficult for any director to satisfy both patients and stockholders, particularly with third-party reimbursements for nursing home care so woefully inadequate.

In all fairness to the administrator of the local nursing home, every attempt was made to provide quality care to the patients. Attempts were even made to admit patients on Medicaid in equal proportion to those paying privately, so that the losses incurred by the institution would be reduced. Long lengths of stay caused an outpour of the patient's personal savings, causing many of the private-fee patients to become eligible for Medicaid reimbursement, which is less than private reimbursement. The profit margin was not what directors expected (although still substantial according to the organization's annual financial report) and so the decision was made to put their investment to work in different services.

The proprietary organization made its decision to close the nursing home over a year before it informed the patients. In fact, it even had enabling legislation introduced into the state legislature as an amendment to a bill that would exempt the organization and its facility from the certificate-of-need process.[27] The sponsored amendment was very specific. It sought waiver of the certificate-of-need process on the condition that the facility was already functioning as a nursing home (under the applicant's management), and the project proposal to convert to a chemical dependency recovery hospital was initiated before the bill was introduced. The certificate-of-need process provides the local community with the opportunity for public hearing to help to determine the need for particular services. Since local health systems agencies had been phased out because of funding cuts 2 years before, the certificate-of-need process is done at the state level. Local input is paramount in the planning process, and California has long been supportive of and sensitive to the specific needs of different communities. However, conduct of the certificate-of-need process at the state level makes getting adequate local input very difficult. The closure of the nursing home and its proposed replacement with a chemical abuse rehabilitation hospital was planned and orchestrated by the vested interests involved. Unfortunately in this case the community was not a part of the planning process.

The county at large is dedicated to providing community-based services. The need for a nursing home in the county far outweighed the need for a chemical dependency recovery hospital. In fact at the time the county had unused beds available for treating drug and alcohol patients, and other sites for the hospital were available in the community. Deciding to locate at one of the other sites would, however, require the organization to go through the certificate-of-need process and the local public hearings. That process takes time, and time is money. Plus there was the risk that another chemical dependency recovery hospital might not be approved.

Before we go on, some explanation should be given of the local control mechanisms. The city has a conditional use permit that it may issue after a series of public hearings indicates that such a permit is warranted. The applicant applies to the city for a conditional use permit to develop a service, such as a skilled nurse facility. The planning department staff analyzes the situation and their report goes before the planning commission, which holds public hearings to permit public discussion. If the planning commission votes in favor of the applicant's request, the permit is granted to the applicant. If not, the applicant can appeal to the city council. The city council has the final word. If appeal is upheld by the city council, a permit is granted; if the appeal is denied, no permit is granted. If application for the permit is denied at any stage, the applicant also has the option of seeking legal council.

The planning process provides the community with a method of determining its own future. In some cases, however, the language in the conditional use permit is not completely clear. In the case of the one issued to the proprietary organization that owned the nursing home, there was a potential for legal argument that the permit would apply equally to a chemical dependency recovery hospital.

The stage is now set to examine the issues that were perceived by the community. They were twofold: first, the community was in dire need of the skilled nursing home beds and, second, the community had been bypassed in the crucial initial planning stages that led to the nursing home's closure. Someone from outside the community was determining just what types of services were needed, effectively denying the community its legal rights.

The citizenry itself wanted desperately to correct this situation. Groups formed to sign petitions, to talk with newspapers, and to try to negotiate with the nursing home's managers for a change of plans. The city council was bombarded by people who wanted to help but did not know what to do. Groups of neighborhood home-owners wanted to have their say, and the family members of patients were irate. In general there was a tremendous amount of energy expended but with little effect.

One group, under the auspices of a religious nonprofit agency (RA), formed a planning committee that approached the nursing home's managers with an offer to sublease the facility. The committee wanted to establish a nonprofit nursing home. To complicate an already difficult situation, the RA's executive director was new. Although she had a strong background in social services and lived in the county, she was not familiar with or known to the network on aging and to the aging community. Thus she was viewed with some suspicion.

Another group (AG) also wanted to approach the nursing home with an alternative of a nonprofit sublease but waited to see what the results of the first negotiations would be. This group had experience in running a nursing home; however, unfortunately there was little communication between the two groups.

A representative of the Grey Panthers, an elderly advocate organization, brought the issue to the monthly meeting of the Commission on Aging asking for assistance and direction. In anticipation of the Commission meeting, Carole Kelly contacted the executive director of the RA and the president of the AG to gather information, to bring it back to the Commission, and to assist the Commission to determine some direction. The information they all provided was helpful in moving toward appropriate decisions and included the following facts. First, the nursing patients were being transferred fairly rapidly. Laws governing transfer require only 30-days' notice, and families were desperately trying to find placement for their members within the county. Although patients have the right to take legal action against being evicted from a facility, families were not willing to expose their loved ones to that type of risk. Most of the patients are severely disabled, old, frail people, and one can certainly understand the families' feelings. The nursing home staff itself, as well as social workers from the county, volunteers, and a consultant group hired by the nursing home, worked hard to find appropriate placement for these patients. One month after the closure was announced, all the patients had been transferred. Many patients were placed in the county but others had to be sent to nursing homes out of the county. Those placed in the northern part of the county might as well have been a thousand miles away. Some of their friends and family members had been able to visit them regularly in the original facility in the southern part of the county. However, because of the facts that friends and family were old themselves, were unable to drive, and lacked public transportation, they now found they could visit only periodically. Thus patients and loved ones were separated. The transferring process itself was traumatic and several patients died. The effects of moving nursing home patients are well documented in the literature.[28-31]

Some decisions were made at the Commission meeting. Carole Kelly was designated as the Commission's representative to the RG's planning committee. The Commission itself would write letters voicing its concern over the nursing home's closure and supporting the attempts being made to acquire the nursing home by a nonprofit agency. These letters would go to the nursing home managers, the RG agency, the local newspapers, and the city council. Commissioners also suggested that the Grey Panthers begin work on legislation that would require a nursing home to allow 90 days after patients had been notified of closure to find a new placement. (This very legislation had been defeated the previous year. It was thought, however, that the political atmosphere was changing and there was a good chance for passage this time around.) The Commission's representative also offered to gather information over the next week and testify before the city council the following Monday.

As the week passed and she spoke with a variety of people, she realized that there were different areas that needed attention. First, there were the community groups who wanted to work with the city. Second, there was the continued discussion between the nonprofit groups and the nursing home's managers. Finally, there was the need for legislation.

The following Monday, she spoke before the city council and basically said,

"People need to get together and here's a number they can call." The Area Agency on Aging (AAA) received calls from interested people, gave out information, and began to put together a list of concerned citizens.

The AG was meeting the following evening and the commissioner spoke briefly with them to get a contact person. She also spoke with others who were concerned. An open community meeting to gather all interested parties seemed appropriate.

By Thursday it was apparent that such a meeting was essential. Several members of the community had been interviewed by the local newspaper, folks were writing letters to the editor, and the newspaper was writing articles on the nursing home industry and the reimbursement industry. The AAA program manager and the commissioner put together a list of people they felt would want to attend a meeting and who could notify others. The commissioner contacted a panel of people who would present information at the meeting, and the notices went out. Arrangements had been made for the meeting to take place in the city hall council chambers.

The panel was to include the commissioner, to do an overview and also describe the Commission; the nursing home administrator, to update the process of the transferring; the executive director of the RG, to describe the negotiations with the nursing home managers; the president of the AG, to present their position; the president of California Homes for the Aged, to talk about possible legislation; and a representative from the Grey Panthers, to speak about their move toward initiating legislation. The nursing home administrator was unable to attend at the last minute but asked the AAA program manager to make his presentation.

The meeting was not as the commissioner had expected. There was a fairly good turnout despite winter storm warnings. About 35 people plus the panel attended. However, emotions ran high. Many of the people had very different agendas. A priest did not understand why the room wasn't packed and wanted to know why everyone he thought should attend had not been informed of the meeting. A physician wanted to know when the panel was planning on building its own nursing home. Others voiced their own concerns about patients, the neighborhood, and other issues.

The panel was able to present most of the information as scheduled and hold a discussion period. When the AAA program manager presented the nursing manager's report, she said she was not acting on behalf of the administrator, but simply said she thought the information should be shared. Patients' family members called the nursing home administrator's information lies. By the time the legislation presentation was given, tempers were hot. The community wanted a solution. A few wanted to know how the panel was going to solve the problem. Finally, the commissioner summarized the presentation and suggested three areas for interested people to address: the community, the negotiations, and the legislation. Someone in the audience suggested that a steering committee be constituted of representatives of groups and consumers. The RG and the AG planned to meet. The commissioner agreed to convene a group interested in introducing legislation. The anger subsided. People grouped together and made plans, and an organized network began to evolve.

We cannot provide an end to this story, since the process goes on. It will take a long time for the outcomes and their consequences to be known. A brief examination of the process follows.

First of all, a steering committee was organized. The chair, who was elected from among the steering committee members, has a background in community organization and is also a member of the community. The committee sees itself as the group that keeps the public aware. The members have initiated a petition-signing movement; they keep in touch with the newspaper and are monitoring the changes in many county institutions. They are ready to mobilize the community when the planning commission hears any application for a conditional use permit. They meet weekly and disseminate information from that meeting through established channels.

The RA is still talking with the nursing home's managers. At one point the RA's executive director arranged a meeting with representatives from the steering committee, other interested agency representatives, the commissioner, and the manager of the new hospital's chemical dependency division. The chemical dependency recovery hospital manager wanted to tell the community about the program. However, the community did not want to hear about it. The manager took back three important facts to the company: (1) the community as a whole was not opposed to chemical dependency rehabilitation programs, (2) the need for nursing home beds was urgent, and (3) the community itself was willing and able to fight for something in which it believed.

The commissioner spent most of her time as a conduit for information. She spoke with several groups, kept the Commission on Aging and the city council informed, and helped keep communication going between the different groups.

She also began working at the legislative level. The community could not do anything about the certificate-of-need waiver, but community members could inform those involved that this type of legislation would not go unnoticed. Staff at the Office of Statewide Health Planning and Development (OSHPD), lobbyists for the cities and towns, health councils, the state ombudsman, and the County Board of Supervisors were advised by the city and the Commission on Aging of the negative impact this waiver legislation had on the local community and asked for closer monitoring of health bills.

Representatives from the Statewide Senior Coalition, the Department of Health and Human Services, the Grey Panthers, consumers, and the Commission on Aging met with the city's assemblyman to look at introducing legislation at the state level that would first give at least 3-months' closure notice to patients and second would provide an opportunity for a management and audit review of an institution if closure was self-initiated. This would be similar to the process that now happens if a state agency initiates closure. At the time of this writing, the bills have been through legislative council and are about to be introduced. The committees mentioned will spend the majority of their energies on the passage of these bills.

The OSHPD is reacting to the interest of the press to the waiver of certificate of need and is reviewing the certificate-of-need exemption that was used to enable closure of the nursing home to take place. There is concern over whether or not the local city requirements for waiver were met before application was made. If not, reversal may be a possibility.

The OSHPD also has asked for local input as to how to prevent the local community from being excluded again in the legislative and permit processes. A simple notification of consumer monitoring is being suggested. If this is instigated, it would prevent special-interest groups from slipping last-minute legislation through without providing time for the democratic process to take place.

The managers of the chemical dependency recovery hospital also plan to apply for a conditional use permit from the city. If they do not and try to operate their hospital without one, the city attorney will file for a court injunction. If they apply for the permit, they will have to go through the public hearing process. If they fail to receive a permit, they have the right to sue (they have hired an attorney), or they may also choose to sublet the facility to some other type of business, which would also have to go through the planning and hearing process. If that fails, the company still has the option of subletting to a nonprofit or another proprietary agency that could run a nursing home if given a permit.

This situation also addresses issues of individual and corporate rights in a capitalistic society. It is very apparent that the community in this example is trying to force a private organization to do what the community wishes. Conditional use permits were developed to enable more local control over community facilities. There is also the issue of the moral responsibility an agency, either nonprofit or proprietary, has to the patients and to the community it serves. It would be possible to engage in extensive arguments over both of these issues; however, the community did not. It made its choice early and is taking the necessary steps to try to implement that choice.

These are not only highly charged political and economic issues but also ethical ones. The retreat of the federal government from regulations to protect people makes them even more pressing.

Commentary

Advocacy is one of the functions of the Commission on Aging. Carole Kelly's initial response as a commissioner to the nursing home closing was based on that advocacy role. It was also based on a feeling that she had a responsibility to the city council that appointed her. She was prepared to be an advocate. What she was not prepared for was the amount of energy and emotion that would be expended not only by her but also by the community at large in dealing with the issue.

Her first real shock came at the informational meeting that she organized. Much of the anger expressed by people at that meeting was directed at the panel, the very panel that was there to help share information and provide direction. In retrospect, it was evident that people needed a forum for venting their anger and frustration. The panel at the informational meeting was possibly seen as the "professional elite" by the community, and obviously there were mixed messages given. The people wanted action; they wanted the panel to act. The panel expected the community to act. Fortunately, although it was a difficult meeting, there was a positive outcome. The commissioner also became aware that first, she needed to be more sensitive to the community and second, although she was known and had credibility among her peers, she had to establish that credibility with other components of the community.

She had the opportunity to do so in the next few weeks as she continued to contact the new chair of the steering committee and the executive director of the RA. She became a resource person to both, since neither were that familiar with the country's network on aging. Her credibility increased in the community by being quoted in the local press. She also wrote letters to the editor clarifying information and relaying messages about what direction the community was taking. She was better prepared for the next meeting with the representative from the chemical dependency recovery hospital. She learned to be assertive through previous community involvement and her nursing background and decided to really use that skill. She presented facts and statistics and countered inferences made by the hospital representatives by bringing attention back to the issues at hand. When the meeting was over, one of the participants told her he liked her much better at this meeting than he had at the informational meeting. Probably one of the reasons was that the agenda was clear to all, and the community had an opportunity to make some progress. The anger had turned to determination and the frustration had turned to planning.

The next month was filled with writing letters, reporting to the city council and Commission on Aging, contacting the OSHPD, gathering a group to meet with the assemblyman to discuss legislation, and speaking before the Chamber of Commerce. What became very apparent was that a fabulous network was being established, and communication was being shared and transferred clearly. Each group recognized the other's expertise and willingly and energetically collaborated on future planning. Strategies are being planned for future planning hearings and for testimony, should the community group be fortunate enough to get the legislation to committee level. The commissioner is also sharing information about the legislative process with the steering committee, using Moorhead's article[32] as a good example of how the process works.

In reviewing the community organization theory and process, the commissioner functioned in a variety of roles. She served as a catalyst, as a collaborator, and as a resource person. She also spent a great deal of time as a conduit for information. She supported her peers, encouraged each group, provided information, and spoke to community agencies and organizations. She defined her role in the beginning as an organizer who would provide information but also who would work in the legislative area. In speaking with fellow commissioners, one thing became apparent. Their interests, skills, and time available were different than hers since most were retired people. Had they been placed in the same situation in which she found herself, they probably would have functioned quite differently.

This process has enabled Carole Kelly to work with others in the community, has enlarged her professional and volunteer network, has given her firsthand experience in community organization, and, hopefully when all is resolved, has helped her provide some safer guarantees that the community in which she lives can continue to give its citizens the type of services that they want and need. The case is an excellent example of Rothman's special planning model of community organization and Ross's inner resources approach to community development.[10,17] It also demonstrates application of Ross's general concept approach in that the Commission on Aging is an advocacy group for issues affecting the elderly. Carole Kelly sought to facilitate the development of a more functional network among agencies working with and for the elderly. Thus she also addressed Ross's process objective of community organization. The experience had been exhausting, exhilarating, frustrating, exciting, and educating. Most of all, it had been worthwhile.

REFERENCES

1. Altshuler, A.A.: Community control: the black demand for participation in large American cities, Indianapolis, Ind., 1970, Pegasus.
2. Turner, J.B., editor: Neighborhood organization for community action, New York, 1968, National Association of Social Workers.
3. National Commission on Community Health Services: Health is a community affair, Cambridge, Mass., 1966, Harvard University Press.
4. Kahn, S.: How people get power: organizing oppressed communities for action, New York, 1970, McGraw-Hill, Inc.
5. Moynihan, D.P.: Maximum feasible misunderstanding: community action in the war on poverty, New York, 1970, The Free Press.
6. Gardner, J.W.: In Common cause: citizen action and how it works, New York, 1972, W.W. Norton & Co., Inc., Publishers.
7. Cox, F.M., and Ahers: Strategies of community organization: a book of readings, ed. 2, Itasca, Ill., 1974, F.E. Peacock Publishers, Inc.
8. Alinsky, S.D.: Rules for radicals: a pragmatic primer for realistic radicals, New York, 1971, Random House.
9. Spergel, I.A.: Community organization: studies in constraint, Beverly Hills, Calif., Sage Publications, Inc., p. 9.
10. Ross, M.G.: Community organization: theory, principles, and practice, ed. 2, New York, 1967, Harper & Row, Publishers, Inc., p. 17.
11. Alinsky, p. 72.
12. Watzlawick, P., Weakland, J.A., and Fisch, R.: Change: principles of problem formation and problem resolution, New York, 1974, W.W. Norton & Co., Publishers.

13. Ross, p. 7-27.
14. Rhoades, R.E.: Peace Corps and the American development philosophy, Human Organization **37**:424-6, 1978.
15. Ross, p. 17.
16. Ross, pp. 24-27.
17. Rothman, J.: Three models of community organization practice. In Cox, F.M., and Ahers, editors: Strategies of community organization: a book of readings, ed. 2, Itasca, Ill., 1974, F.E. Peacock, pp. 22-39.
18. Chin, R., and Benne, K.D.: General strategies for effecting changes in human systems. In Bennis, W.G., and others, editors: The planning of change, ed. 3, New York, 1976, Holt, Rinhart, & Winston, Inc., pp. 22-45.
19. Watzlawick, pp. 24-27.
20. Freire, P.: Pedagogy of the oppressed, New York, 1981, The Continuum Publishing Corp.
21. Freire, P.: Education for critical consciousness, New York, 1981, The Continuum Publishing Corp.
22. Coover, V., Deacon, E., Esser, C., and Moore, C.: Resource manual for a living revolution, ed. 2, Philadelphia, Penn., 1978, Movement for a New Society, pp. 140-150.
23. Ross, pp. 203-231.
24. Lurie, H.L.: The community organization method in social work education. In The Curriculum Study, New York, 1959, Council on Social Work Education.
25. Hersey, P., and Blanchard, K.H.: Management of organizational behavior: utilizing human resources, ed. 3, Englewood Cliffs, N.J., 1977, Prentice-Hall, Inc.
26. Fottler, M.D., Smith, H.L., and James, W.L.: Profits and patient care quality in nursing homes: are they compatible? The Gerontologist **21**:532, 1981.
27. Johnson, R.: Health planning (SB 637, Chapter 869), sections 437.112 and 437.114, 1981, California State Health and Safety Code.
28. Borup, J.H.: Relocation: attitudes, information network, and problems encountered, The Gerontologist **21**:501, 1981.
29. Brody, E., Kleban, M., and Moss, M.: Measuring the impact of change, The Gerontologist **14**:299, 1974.
30. Schulz, R., and Brenner, G.: Relocation of the aged: a review and theoretical analysis, Journal of Gerontology **32**:323, 1977.
31. Cohen, E.S.: Legal issues in "transfer trauma" and their impact, The Gerontologist **21**:520, 1980.
32. Moorhead, J.: Community health nurses' involvement in legislative processes. In Archer, S.E., and Fleshman, R., editors: Community health nursing: patterns and practice, ed. 2, North Scituate, Mass., 1979, Duxbury Press.

4

CONSULTATION PROCESS

Conceptions of what consultants can do range from expecting them to be able to do everything to assuming that they are useless. Somewhere in between these extremes is the reality for most consultants.

The title *consultant* connotes a certain air of dignity; it denotes a set of skills in a specific area or process and hints at expertise in a particular field. Consultation is practiced in many settings, such as communities, schools, and business organizations, and by many types of human service workers, such as community organizers, psychologists, nurses, and educators, who may or may not have had formal preparation in consultation.

Here we discuss the consultation process, ethical dilemmas, and marketing techniques to assist you in developing consulting skills. The model we use for the process is described by Lippitt and Lippitt in *The Consulting Process in Action.*[1] These authors focus on consultation as a collaborative helping process whether in planned change or in evaluation. This basic philosophy intertwines comfortably with our systems theory framework and our emphasis on collaboration in community change. We refer to the consultant system as the *consultant* and the target community system as the *consultee* throughout this chapter. The collaborative intersystem is where consultant and consultee meet and work together toward the desired outcomes. At some point we are all members of that collaborative intersystem.

OVERVIEW OF CONSULTATION

Consultation has been considered an umbrella label for many variations of professional practices such as teaching, supervising, and caring, all of which have bases in interpersonal processes.[2] The numerous definitions of consultation reflect these variations and are related to differences in the consultant's preparation and frame of reference. For example, in the field of mental health, Caplan,[3] Norman and Forti,[4] and Mannino and others[5] place high priority on the interpersonal relationship between the consultant and the consultee. In organizational development, Lippitt and Lippitt[1] and, in nursing, Deloughery and others[6] describe an orderly process to bring about change. Gibb's[7] process of working with groups stresses data gathering.

Croley,[8] in international development, also emphasizes the process specifically for the purpose of the transfer of knowledge and skills in problem solving.

An analysis of the various existing definitions of consultation identifies the following basic components:

1. A process involving continual progression through a number of stages from a beginning to a defined end
2. A data-gathering enterprise in which needs are identified and actions are taken based on the most current appraisal of available data and cycled feedback
3. A vehicle for assistance in the various forms of insight, understanding, knowledge and skill transfer, institution building, and systems change
4. An interpersonal relationship between two or more people or systems, each assuming specific roles and each affecting and being affected by the other
5. A voluntary arrangement in which the consultant has no administrative responsibility for the consultee or for implementing recommendations, and the consultee has the freedom to accept, modify, or reject the consultant's contributions

Common themes that are particularly relevant to our conceptualization of collaborative consultation include an exchange process for the giving and receiving of knowledge and skills, interpersonal interactions, and an equitable relationship between the consultant and the consultee.

The diversity in consultation definitions and practices may have impeded the development of generally accepted consultation models and theoretical approaches. Even in the field of mental health, in which significant theoretical work was begun by Caplan[3] on consultee-, client-, and program-centered approaches and in which consultation has been used extensively to provide community outreach and education services as one of the five basic components of community mental health center programs, this lack of progress has led Mannino[5] to conclude that consultation practices are dominated by common-sense approaches so that strategies vary from one consultant to another.

The use of consultation is expanding. As a result, numerous articles are appearing in the consultation literature based on personal experiences and impressions (cited examples provide an illustrative rather than an exhaustive review).[9-18] There are few theoretical models that are clearly defined—conceptually, attitudinally, and behaviorally—so that one model can be distinguished from another. Dworkin and Dworkin[19] provide an example of an attempt to clarify through comparative analysis four currently popular consultation models: Caplan's consultee-centered model, Lippitt and Lippitt's group process model, Alinsky's social action model, and Kelly's ecological model. This analysis illustrates differences among the models in the way consultation is defined, in the consultant's perceptions of her or his own role and that of the target population, in the goals of consultation, and in evaluation techniques.

For example, because of the highly personal nature of Caplan's consultee-centered approach, in which the consultant is expected to improve the consultee's insight into the problems of the consultee's client, objective evaluation techniques have been difficult to develop and implement. The outcomes of Alinsky's social action model, in which the consultant as political strategist seeks to transfer power to the oppressed constituency, are best validated by the evidence of the emergence of indigenous leadership. The application of these models influences not only the strategies a consultant uses and the relationships she or he develops but also the particular consequences in terms of benefits and costs for the people affected by the outcomes.

The call for greater conceptual clarity is not intended to limit the consultant's choices of available models and strategies. Rather this improved clarity would facilitate the consultant's awareness of her or his own preferred model or style. A major advantage of this awareness is the consultant's ability to communicate clearly how and what she or he is prepared to offer to prospective employers and consultees.

Research on consultation practice is another impetus for greater specificity of consultation models. Existing research findings are difficult to compare because of the inconsistent terminology, the lack of behavioral specificity of the consultation strategies used in the studies, and the differences in measurement methods.[20] Beginning efforts to define the current consultation models suggest that these models can be made conceptually and behaviorally distinct. Clear specification of the models would facilitate research efforts to determine if the processes and outcomes of the consultation actually reflect what the models depict and to test the differential effectiveness of the models in bringing about desired outcomes.

Despite the extensive use of consultation and its acknowledged effectiveness, another deficit is the dearth of published consultation research and evaluation.[21] Little is understood about the dynamics of consultant-consultee relationships, that is, how they develop, change, or stay the same during consultation; the impact of particular consulting strategies on the overall consultation; or the contextual variables that influence process, outcome, and consequences.[22-28] Such research would promote empirically valid decisions about which theoretical and practical consultation approaches are likely to be most effective in bringing about the desired change. Shrinking budgets in many health and human services organizations increase the needs of employers to have much more empirical information on consultation to enable them to use their limited resources most effectively.

CONSULTATION ROLES

The consultant plays multiple roles during a consultation process. These roles range from more nondirective ones, such as objective observer and process counselor, to more directive ones, such as expert and advocate.[29] The question for the consultant to answer in selecting roles is not which single role to take throughout the consultation process but rather when, how, and to what degree to play one or all of a variety of roles. Choices depend on her or his own personal and theoretical preferences, what has and has not worked before, the nature of the consultee's initial request, the norms and standards of the consultee system, and other contextual factors.[29] The overriding ground rule for consultants is to select consultant roles that will eventually help to create collaborative relationships.

However, the very fact that collaboration is a shared process means that one may not always be able to play consultant roles that foster her or his particular view of collaborative planning for change. Consultees may have very different expectations for the roles of the consultant. They may have highly specific time-limited needs and may want the consultant to play a task-oriented and directive role to get the job done for them. The consultant who values collaboration can either adapt her or his style to fit the consultee's expressed demand or decline the contract. On the other hand, consultees at the outset of the consultation may not have a clear image of what collaborative planning is because of past experiences with different consultants' styles. For example, they may expect, based on experience, that all consultants are information experts who have *the* answer. The consultant and consultees, then, need the opportunity to discuss and negotiate how they will work together, what roles they will play, and how they will monitor and negotiate further role and relationship changes as needed throughout the consultation. All must be responsive and willing to change as necessary. Determining how much collaboration is possible is in fact a collaborative exercise in itself.

The point of entry influences both subsequent role relationships and the eventual outcome of consultation. The mode of entry often determines whose agent the consultant becomes. For example, the consultation process may be initiated by a third party who sponsors the consultation but who does not actively participate. However, if this third party has administrative responsibility for those who must work together, it retains power to influence the process and what eventually happens as a result of the consultation. To attempt to avoid being cast as either the hired hand of the third party or the agent of the actual consultees, the consultant may choose to negotiate exchange relationships so that there is give and take among all participants. Thus the consultant, consultees, and third party all share power and control of the process, outcome, and long-term consequences of the consultation.[30]

The influences on consultant and consultee roles and relationships are made even more complex when we add the consideration of cultural differences to the list. The beliefs, values, norms, and traditions that are part of one's national and ethnic heritage permeate every aspect of life; how one perceives and interprets experiences, communicates, relates to others, and behaves in all kinds of circumstances.[31]

Consultants may be more acutely aware of actual and potential conflicts caused by cultural differences because of experiences in international consultation situations. The impact of culture on role relationships is not merely because of exotic differences in customs and traditional practices, communication problems, or personality conflicts. The impact is greatly influenced by the altered emphases on the basic and dominant values and norms that govern roles, status definitions, and symbolic systems that give meaning and predictability to human interactions and communications.[32-36] However, these cultural conflicts can be effectively addressed once they are recognized, as Sally Bisch's experience demonstrates.

Recently Sally Bisch was a consultant for a health agency that provided consultants to assist national nurses to strengthen nursing curriculums and to prepare programs. By the standards in the country where she was consulting, she was considered young for her position and its inherent status. She was also a female foreign nurse. As part of her assignment, she periodically had to report to the director of a government department, a senior male physician. According to the customs in that country, a young female nurse would automatically defer to his seniority and authority. But because she was an international consultant, she was expected to offer advice and recommendations to the director about proposals that were critical to the continued development of nursing programs in the country. When the role and status conflicts between the consultant and the director became uncomfortably clear in a meeting, the consultant and her national counterparts, who were senior nurses in the government, devised strategic ways to minimize her leadership role at the next meeting, at which time they would present their major proposal again. It was agreed that the next meeting should be conducted in the national language rather than in English. They prepared a statement written in their language and in English of the nursing program's needs, goals, and resource requirements; what had been accomplished through the collaborative efforts of the consultant and her national counterparts; and what still needed to be done to bring about the desired outcome. They also sought to strengthen the proposal's legitimacy and enhance its potential for acceptance by inviting a senior male physician whom they knew supported the proposal to come to the next meeting and speak in its favor.

The strategy worked. In reviewing the results of the meeting, the consultant and her nurse counterparts were convinced that their proposal's support by a senior male physician greatly contributed to the director's decision to approve it as submitted. They had watched the director and the other physician confer on the proposal's pros and cons and clarify numerous misunderstandings the director had had. They realized they had been successful in minimizing the role and status conflict between the young nurse consultant and the director that had interfered with the director's acceptance of the proposal when it was first presented by the consultant.

This example illustrates the consultant's use of the collaborative process in working with her counterparts to find strategies that would resolve the role and status dilemma between her and the director. The most important consideration in this situation was to get the proposal approved even if it meant that the spokesman for nursing was a physician, not a nurse.

This example also illustrates that in addition to a consultant's need to be aware of the consultee's cultural value system and its impact on the consultation process, she or he needs to be aware of her or his own professional and cultural value systems and their impact on practice. Masson[37] advises nurses who are considering international work to answer two questions for themselves: "What professional values . . . would I be willing to adapt or set aside (and) what values . . . would I refuse to compromise?" In Sally Bisch's case, as a nurse from the United States where nursing is a relatively autonomous profession, she had to answer for herself the question, "How comfortable am I in having a nonnurse speak for nursing given the circumstances in which I am working?" Her personal decision was that it was acceptable to her since neither she nor her female nurse counterparts could be nearly as effective in this situation as could their male physician colleague. The consultant and her nurse counterparts discussed the situation and their beliefs and values and together reached consensus that the physician should be their spokesman. For all of them, the end of having their proposal approved justified the needed means.

What we have said about cultural differences is as applicable in the United States as it is in other countries and cultures. A consultant may live in the same country as do her or his consultees, but that fact does not mean that they all live according to the same cultural and other values, norms, and standards. Because the United States is culturally pluralistic, a consultant must be sensitive to and respectful of cultural differences and take these differences into account when she or he consults with culturally diverse groups.

There is much in the consultation literature about the pros and cons of consultants from inside compared to consultants from outside the client system. Our model of a collaborative intersystem largely obviates the significance of this issue. However, we do describe some insider-outsider considerations in Table 5-3, p. 97.

CONSULTATION PROCESS

Lippitt and Lippitt's process of consultation, which provides the organizing framework for this chapter, is based on their concept of consultation as "a two way interaction—a process of seeking, giving, and receiving help. [It] is aimed at aiding a person, group, organization, or larger system in mobilizing internal and external resources to deal with problem confrontation and change efforts."[38]

Basically this interaction process involves three main phases: initiation, problem solving, and termination. Lippitt and Lippitt[38] stress that consultation is a reciprocal interpersonal process that occurs between and among the people who participate in the process and who draw on available resources to bring about change. Interpersonal relationships between the consultant and the consultees in the collaborative intersystem are critical ingredients in consultation because they not only facilitate the final outcome of the consultation process but also promote mutual change and reward as all participants in consultation share and learn together.

> Too frequently clients in their frantic search for a solution, and consultants, in their drive to demonstrate their expertise, pass each other in the night without realizing that at the root of giving and receiving help is the richness of human encounter.[39]

There also is an intrapersonal process in consultation that is often less obvious because it takes place outside the observable interactions between and among participants.[40] Both consultant and consultees go through individual preparations for the consultation situation. In their own personal ways they internally analyze the interactions, the data, and the planning and evaluation activities of which they are a part. Each one reaches her or his positions based on personal interests, experiences, and interpretations. Although one cannot know what these intrapersonal processes are nor when they take place, one must be aware that they are an integral part of consultation for all of the participants.

Lippitt and Lippitt[41] identify the following six phases in the consultation process:

1. Initial contact or entry
2. Formulating a contract and establishing a helping relationship
3. Problem identification and diagnostic analysis
4. Setting goals and planning for action
5. Taking action and cycling feedback
6. Contract completion: continuity, support, and termination

According to their definition, the implementation of these phases enables the consultant and consultees to deal with change efforts. Consultation and change are not dissimilar processes, as Table 4-1 shows.

TABLE 4-1

Comparison of nursing process, planned change, and consultation

Nursing process	Planned change	Consultative process
Assessment	Development of a need for change	Initial contact and entry
	Establishment of a change relationship	Formulating a contract and establishing a helping relationship
Diagnosis	Working toward change —diagnosis of problem	Problem identification and diagnostic analysis
Implementation	—establishing goals and intentions of actions	Goal setting and planning Taking action and
Evaluation	Generalization and stability of change —evaluation	Cycling feedback
	Achieving a terminal relationship	Contract completion, continuity, support, termination

From Oda, D.S.: Nursing Leadership 5:7-9, March 1982. Reprinted with permission of the publisher.

Nurses, planners, community organizers, ministers, lawyers, and a multitude of volunteers in the community may be more familiar with the cyclic process of planned change. Should you not be, please see Chapter 2. As this comparison demonstrates, we are going through virtually the same process even though we may be using different labels.

A step-by-step review of Lippitt and Lippitt's consultation process[1] follows.

Step 1: initial contact and entry

Consultation situations arise when a consultee seeks help, a consultant offers to help, or a third party who recognizes the need for change brings the consultee and the consultant together. The initial contact may be very easy if the consultant is or has been a part of the consultee system or has done previous consultative work with it. For example, two of us have done serial consultation internationally. Each time we go back to the same setting, reentry is facilitated by the fact that we already know our counterparts and have some experience in the system that can be used in undertaking the consultation task on each subsequent visit. This serial consultation also enables members of the collaborative intersystem to build on and make adjustments in work that they have previously accomplished together.

Consultants who come into contact with a consultee system for the first time bring with them an objectivity that will be very useful in the consultation process. They will have a great deal to learn about the consultee system with which they will work. Much of this information can be gained as part of the functions within the collaborative intersystem and be a relatively nonthreatening vehicle for developing the kind of support that is needed before real collaboration can occur.

Clear communication is essential throughout the consultative process but never more so than at this initial step. Consultant and consultee must be in agreement on their understanding of the need for and at least some notion of the overall goal that the consultant is to assist the consultee system to achieve. This is not the detailed goal-setting process discussed in Chapter 2 but rather an introductory approach to goals that must take place to determine whether the consultant has the expertise that may be of assistance to the consultee system. Consultants should do the best they can to get a valid feel for the consultee system's grasp of its needs and its willingness to work with the consultant to address them as effectively as possible.

We have already discussed how the consultant's point of entry into the consultative situation can lead to confusion as to whose agent the consultant really is. As with all entrees, one has only one chance to make first impressions; much thought should be given to the way in which the kind of first impression that will best aid the ensuing collaborative process is made.

This is an exploratory time. In some cases, screening committees are established to interview potential consultants and to be interviewed by them. It is a time when both the consultant and the consultee are free to ask questions of each other to determine their future together. It is step one in the collaborative process.

Step 2: formulating a contract and establishing a helping relationship

Agreeing on a contract and putting it in writing serves two purposes: it establishes the framework for the process, and it is a legal and binding contract between the consultant and the consultee. Expected outcomes, time commitments, financial arrangements, accountability of the consultant, what type of support the consultee will receive, where activities will take place, and items such as working space and clerical support must be included. Mechanisms to ensure that the collaborative intersystem will receive feedback at stipulated intervals must be built in. Since financial considerations are given at this time, a time line for the consultation services should be very clear. Consultants must realistically plan the time frame or they may find that they are working on a project after the money runs out.

Step 3: problem identification and diagnostic analysis

Meetings to clarify the problem and orient the consultant to its dimensions occur at this stage. Together the members of the collaborative intersystem identify the driving and restraining forces in the situation. A forcefield analysis such as that shown in Fig. 4 serves as a visualization of the variables in the situation that plans

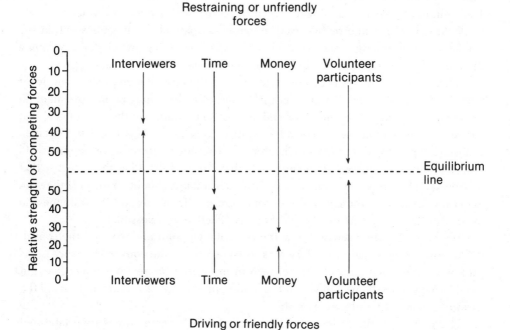

FIG. 4
Lewin's forcefield analysis applied to decisions in senior resources survey.

must address.[42] This is also the time when the group explores the available data on the problem and decides what other information, if any, must be obtained and how to obtain it.

Together the members of the collaborative intersystem define the functions of each member and continue to ensure communication and feedback. The consultant will have to adjust her or his consultation style to the expectations of the group at least to some extent, while continuing to help them to be more comfortable with a developing collaborative relationship.

Step 4: goal setting and planning

Processes and methods for dealing with this step of the consultation process are discussed in detail in Chapter 2.

Step 5: taking action and cycling feedback

Lippitt and Lippitt[43] state that "a major motivation for continuing effort comes from frequent experiences of successful movement on a defined path that leads somewhere." If the time line has been clearly drawn and the steps in the process have been identified along with the goals, the structure is in place to evaluate accomplishments and to give positive feedback. PERT, presented in Figure 3 (p. 34), and the time line in Figure 7 (p. 173) are methods to identify the necessary steps in the process.

Step 6: contract completion: continuity, support, and termination

The report of findings and recommendations should be completed as stipulated in the contract. Although consultation as we view it is a collaborative endeavor, the ultimate responsibility and accountability for decisions and their outcomes and consequences belongs to the consultee system. The collaborative intersystem reports its findings and recommendations. The consultee system has the final choice of whether or not and how to implement these recommendations.

The consultant and the consultee should also review the original contract to evaluate the success of the relationship and to allow the consultee and the consultant the opportunity to evaluate everyone's performance.

Hopefully, the relationship between the consultant and the consultee is successful; the results would be a resolution of the consultee's problem through a mutually beneficial collaborative process.

EXAMPLE OF THE CONSULTATION PROCESS

This consultation process as described can be used for community evaluations particularly on a contractual, short-term basis. Briefly, here is the process that was used from the consultants' viewpoint in conducting the senior resources survey, the evaluation example in Chapter 8.

Step 1: initial contact and entry

Sarah Archer was serving as an officer of a county Commission on Aging (COA). She was also teaching at the School of Nursing of the University of California at San Francisco and was preparing to teach community assessment and organization classes, for which she needed field placements. The program manager of the Area Agency on Aging (AAA) was in need of baseline data for future planning. The AAA had very little money. Here were two people who saw that they might be able to assist each other. We developed a plan that involved the AAA contracting with her to conduct a baseline resource survey of seniors in the county that also enabled the instructor to offer a realistic learning experience for students. Both the AAA and the School of Nursing were winners in this arrangement. This facilitated entry.

Sarah Archer had the advantage of knowing the target community system and already having credibility because of her role on the COA. At this time Carole Kelly was a graduate student and would be a teaching assistant in the upcoming courses. She also was familiar with the county and the people who would be involved in the project. Both the instructor and the teaching assistant believed they could work effectively with the AAA program manager and with the community agencies that would become involved. The AAA program manager also was comfortable with them, since we had all worked together for years.

Step 2: formulating a contract and establishing a helping relationship

Following these preliminary discussions, a contract for the senior resources survey was written. The time line (see Fig. 7, p. 173) was tightly drawn to conform to the University's calendar. Carole Kelly would develop and pretest the instrument in the fall quarter. During the winter quarter, Sarah Archer and Carole Kelly would plan and develop the community assessment course, which was to be taught for the first time in the spring quarter to 39 undergraduate students, and revise the community organization course that would be offered concurrently to graduate students in community health nursing. They would also work closely with the AAA staff as well as with other agencies in the community to obtain an adequate sample of volunteer older persons to be surveyed in the spring quarter, when the courses would be taught and the survey would be actually conducted.

The instructor and assistant, as members of the evaluator system, and the AAA program manager and her planner, as members of the community system, created the collaborative intersystem in which the actual interaction occurred. Because of the long-time association of the members of the representatives of the two systems, the collaborative intersystem very quickly took on a life of its own that was separate from the systems that evaluators and agency executives represented. The process and outcomes of this collaboration were very rewarding.

Step 3: problem identification and diagnostic analysis

Discussions at meetings centered around driving and restraining forces for doing the survey.[42] Obviously, money and time were restraining forces. Having enough interviewers was a driving force (at least it was seen that way at that time). Later, it was believed that having so many interviewers could also be seen as a restraining force (see Fig. 7, p. 173, and Chapter 8).

The evaluators and the AAA worked closely together to develop the survey instrument. It was important to ask the questions that would give the baseline data desired. The AAA manager was also familiar with the areas where general information was lacking about the elderly and was willing to spend time helping to ensure the validity of the interview schedule.

Step 4: goal setting and planning

The overall goal of the survey was to provide baseline data to the AAA by the end of the following summer. A time line was established that showed the milestone events such as getting the protocol approved by the university's human research committee, publicizing the survey in the community and asking for volunteer participants, developing the class, training the interviewers, doing the survey, analyzing the data, and reporting the results, both in written and verbal form. The time line is in Fig. 7, p. 173. All members, therefore, knew exactly what had to be done by when and by whom.

Step 5: taking action and cycling feedback

The process involved constant interaction among members of the collaborative intersystem to validate the interview schedule and report on the progress. The relationship between AAA and the evaluators continued to be open and responsive, and feedback was solicited regularly. The opportunity to discuss problems or changes was always there and was used frequently. All participants expressed feelings of success along the way.

The volunteer subjects were contacted, the students were trained, the interviews were completed, the data were analyzed, and the information was put together for presentation. This process is discussed in detail in Chapter 8 and the final report and data are included.

Step 6: contract completion: continuity, support, and termination

The contract was completed when Carole Kelly presented the oral reports to the COA and AAA and the evaluators sent the written report to the AAA. The material that was gathered was used for future planning and provided the AAA with some badly needed baseline information. The process proved to be a valuable field experience for graduate and undergraduate students.

ETHICAL CONSIDERATIONS IN THE CONSULTATION PROCESS

In consulting activities with aggregates and communities for planning and evaluating change efforts, consultants collaborate in making choices that involve technical and value judgments. In making technical judgments, consultants ask if the choice is feasible, effective, efficient, reliable, valid, and so on. In making value judgments, consultants ask if the choice is good, right, worthy, acceptable, just, or fair.[44]

Issues, particularly ethical ones, arise because of the differences and disagreements in value judgments and the resulting decisions. We discuss to some extent the issues involving value judgments concerning the goals and actions of plans in Chapter 2, in which we are particularly concerned that the resulting outcomes do not have intended or unintended detrimental consequences for the people most affected by the changes that are planned. In Chapter 5 we discuss the ethical issues surrounding participation in evaluation. Here we confine our discussion to the ethical considerations involved in the value judgments consultants make in deciding how they behave and how they collaborate with the community system in the consultation process.

Ethics is the branch of philosophy that concerns itself with questions of human conduct. When one makes judgments about other people's behavior being good or bad or right or wrong, one is using a set of ethical rules or standards to guide judgments. Consultants not only abide by a set of personal and societal ethical rules, but as professionals who are concerned with the quality of the service that we provide, we adhere to our own professional group's code of conduct. By the enforcement of these codes, professions can guarantee to the society they serve that their practitioners are not only competent but ethical. These codes of ethics provide standards for guidance of a consultant's behavior as well as safeguards for the community members with whom she or he collaborates and standards for use in the evaluation of the consultant's behavior.[45]

The consultation profession, particularly in the social and behavioral sciences, has not achieved the stature and unity to develop or enforce a widely accepted code of conduct.[44] Lippitt and Lippitt, in their review of several different codes of ethics, select eight items from the American Society for Training and Development Code of Ethics· that refer specifically to consultant-consultee relationships.[46] Consultants shall:

1. Not conduct activities that may cause any colleague or training participant unnecessary embarrassment or disparagement
2. Not violate confidences or break promises, unless the disclosure of confidential information serves professional purposes or is required by law
3. Limit their activities as facilitators of change to functions for which they have been adequately trained and abstain particularly from areas of psychological activity for which they have no professional qualifications

4. Not knowingly distort or misrepresent facts concerning training and development activities to any individual, organization, or employer
5. Openly share information and data that will advance the state of the professional art
6. Maintain a professional attitude toward the introduction of new knowledge in the field of training and development
7. Recognize the desire of individuals and organizations to improve themselves and permit no exploitation of this desire by unethical use of the profession or of its members
8. Recognize that society in general accords status to consultants, and that in return they have an obligation to serve the needs of society

This list includes protection not only for the consultee system in the immediate situation but also for the consultation profession as a whole, since a consultant's behavior is a reflection on her or his professional association. However, we believe that the most important consideration for service-oriented professionals should be the ultimate welfare of the aggregates and communities with whom we consult. The most basic tool in consultation work is the relationship that is established with consultees. It must be based on mutual trust and respect. To that end consultants must relate in ways that convey trustworthiness, openness, honesty, integrity, empathy, flexibility, and so on.

Some questions that we consultants might ask ourselves as a means of using our own personal and professional standards in our consultation work are:

1. Do I have the necessary expertise and skills for the specific assignment?
2. Am I giving an honest representation of my credentials?
3. Am I aware of my own views and biases and their potential impact on how I relate with others?
4. Is there a conflict of interest on my part?
5. Do I think I can work with the parameters of my responsibilities and the existing circumstances?
6. Can I be flexible enough in adapting my style to what the consultees want?
7. Can I obtain adequate social support outside of the consultation situation?
8. Am I capable of the tact and discretion this assignment requires?

These questions do not comprise an exhaustive list. No doubt others can be added. The point is that we consultants need to continue to examine and clarify our own ethical standards ourselves and with the assistance of our professional colleagues. As is the case with many other topics in this book, ethical standards do not remain constant but also change over time through reflections on new and different consultation experiences.

A set of interrelated considerations are critical to collaborative consultant-consultee relationships. These are the actual or perceived power of the consultant and

the actual or perceived freedom of the consultee to participate fully in the consultation process.[47] We have alluded to these considerations in previous discussions in this
chapter and in Chapter 2. We believe that they are so important that they deserve
repeated attention. We as consultants bring considerable knowledge, experience,
and skills to the consultation process. We need to be aware that our perceived expertise, evidenced by the fact that we have been brought in to "help with or to solve
a problem," and the accompanying image trappings, such as titles, resumes, and
business cards, are a setup for power differentials and social distance barriers between consultants and consultees. Unequal power relationships are unfortunately
usually stacked against the consultees, particularly those who because of inadequate
experience or knowledge are not likely to be in positions to enter immediately into
equitable relationships. When faced with consultants whom they perceive to have
considerable power and status, these consultees may feel constrained to accept the
consultant's recommendations even if not appropriate rather than to appear disre-
spectful or risk disapproval if they openly reject or seek to modify them. The un-
fortunate result is that the consultees do not receive the assistance they sought and
paid for, and subsequently remain in their same subordinate state, still facing their
problem. This picture may be an extreme one. However, even the slightest infringement on the consultees' right to participate and make decisions freely is intolerable,
particularly for those consultants who seek to work collaboratively with consultee
systems.[48]

The initial circumstances may foster power differentials, but it is the consultants'
responsibility to do something about them. We must consciously and consistently
enable the consultees to speak for their own interests by helping them to make use of
their own abilities effectively, to realize their potential strengths, and to obtain
information and skills to get and use power.[49] In a sense, consultants are promoting
second-order change in the very structure of the consultation relationships in which
we are involved. We are trying to change the rules of the system by empowering
the consultees with whom we work so that the consultees end up with at least equal
if not more power than the consultants. Consultants will know that the consultation
has had at least one successful outcome when consultees say, "We did it ourselves."

MARKETING CONSULTATION SKILLS

There is a growing need for consultation services. Many communities, aggregates, and organizations find themselves facing new or more complex situations.
Their permanent staff often do not have the specific expertise to evaluate and plan
ways to effectively address these situations. Thus a consultant is sought as a means for
getting the kinds of ad hoc help that are needed. This approach to one-time-only or
very specific needs can be highly cost-effective, even though the initial expenditure
for the consultant's services may seem high.

In the long run, assuming that the consultant and consultees can reach a consensus on what should be done to address the specific situation, the consultees get the benefit of the consultant's expertise for a short time without having to create a regular position for and to retain the consultant beyond the time that her or his services are most needed. In planning budgets, therefore, the creation of a substantially funded line item for outside consultation as needed can be a very sound fiscal management practice.

Knowing that the market is potentially available and that you have the skills to meet many prospective consultees' needs is reassuring. It is not, however, enough. You must let prospective clients know what your skills are and that you are available. Marketing is your best approach.[50-52] The following are some ways in which marketing can be done.

Networking

Many of you are members of a number of professional networks in which you have the opportunity to get to know colleagues with whom you may someday work collaboratively as consultants and consultees. Thus, very often you already know and are known to your counterparts before someone initiates a consultative situation. Indeed, these professional networks offer invaluable opportunities for consultants to meet others, to learn about others' skills and interests, and to tell them about their own. When one or another member of the network needs assistance at a later time, she or he will have a good idea on whom to call for that help. Under these circumstances, you will find that much of the initial contact with collaborative potential is already established.

Use of written resumes

A consultant must remain aware of opportunities at work or through voluntary situations where one can apply for a consulting position. When you see that a consultant is wanted and you feel that your skills are appropriate, send a resume to the agency. Be sure to list your voluntary consulting jobs in the resume. Agencies are looking for experience, not whether you were paid for service. Remember that your first impression, which you want to be a good one, will be made through your resume. Make sure that it conveys a positive image of you and your abilities. If you do not know how to prepare a resume, get help.[52]

Advertisements

Many consultants begin to branch out into community agencies by advertising their skills. This can be done through local newspapers, professional journals, and community announcements. The best advertisements are by word of mouth from satisfied consultees, especially in a closely knit community.

Volunteering

One of the ways to establish your credibility as a consultant is to volunteer your services, especially to organizations for whom you would like to work. Start out by working with others or limiting your initial undertakings to the areas in which you are most comfortable. This method gives you visibility and also the opportunity to control the amount of work you undertake. You can do this within your work setting as well as in professional and community organizations. Volunteers with skills are much appreciated in this day and age in which money is scarce and needs are many. Volunteering can also give you an opportunity to acquire or to perfect skills in many areas that you can market later.

Professional cards

Many consultants carry professional cards that state the agencies and positions with which they are affiliated. Your areas of consultation availability can be added to those cards and as you distribute them, you can describe the kind of consulting you do. This is always a good method to use in expanding your network.

Initiating consulting positions

This is an innovative way of developing a consulting practice. Recognizing needs within a community setting or agency, contacting the powers that be, and perhaps even developing your own form of income through grants or delegated funding are ways to establish a consultative practice. The need for consultants always exists, and it is a wonderful bonus if the consultant has her or his own funding resources as well as expertise.

Setting fees

Many professionals in the field of health and human services do consulting as an adjunct to their regular positions. They are comfortable with this type of arrangement especially since it has the added incentive of extra pay. It is important for prospective consultants to check out the competitive rates for the type of service they are offering. If an agency is advertising for a consultant, cost has already been considered, and so the consultant and the agency should be prepared to negotiate. If the consultant is working full time in another position, time will have to be negotiated. This is all part of selling your services to the market.

SUMMARY

In this chapter we have discussed consultation from a collaborative perspective, stressing the need for the consultant and the consultee to work together toward the objectives of the consultation process. Consultation roles were explored with a particular view to strategies to deal effectively with power and status differences. Several examples of the consultation process show the steps involved from initial contact to completion of the consultation report and termination. We conclude with some thoughts on the ethics of consultation and some ideas on how you can market your consulting skills more effectively.

REFERENCES

1. Lippitt, G., and Lippitt, R.: The consulting process in action, LaJolla, Calif., 1978, University Associates, Inc.
2. Lippitt, R.: Dimensions of the consultant's job, The Journal of Social Issues 15(2):5-12, 1959.
3. Caplan, G.: The theory and practice of mental health consultation, New York, 1970, Basic Books, Inc, Publishers.
4. Norman, E.C., and Forti, T.J.: A study of the process and outcome of mental health consultation, Community Mental Health Journal 8:261-270, November 1972.
5. Mannino, F.V., and others: The practice of mental health consultation, DHEW Publication no. 74-112, Washington, D.C., 1975, Department of Health, Education, and Welfare.
6. Deloughery, G., Gebbie, K., and Newman, B.: Consultation and community organization in community mental health nursing, Baltimore, 1971, The Williams & Wilkins Co., pp. 53-74.
7. Gibbs, J.R.: The role of the consultant, The Journal of Social Issues 15(2):1-4, 1959.
8. Croley, H.T.: Roles of international advisors, Health Education Monographs 3:362-371, Fall 1975.
9. Blake, P.: The clinical specialist as nurse consultant, Journal of Nursing Administration 7:33-36, December 1971.
10. Bloch, H.S.: Experiences in establishing school consultation, American Journal of Psychiatry 129:63-68, July 1972.
11. Hansen, J.C.: Prevention through teacher consultation, Journal of School Health 47:289-292, May 1977.
12. Musante, G., and Gallemore, J.L.: Utilization of a staff development group in prison consultation, Community Mental Health Journal 9:224-232, Fall 1973.
13. Peterson, C.L.: Consultation with community care systems, Social Work in Health Care 2:181-191, Winter 1976-77.
14. Sedgewick, R.: The role of the process consultant, Nursing Outlook 21:773-775, December 1973.
15. Signell, K., and Scott, P.A.: Mental health consultation: an interaction model, Community Mental Health Journal 7:288-302, December 1971.
16. Termini, M., and Ciechoski, M.A.: The consultation process, Issues in Mental Health Nursing 3:77-88, 1981.
17. Nuckolls, K.B.: The consultation process: a reciprocal relationship, Maternal Child Nursing 2:11-16, 1977.
18. Severin, N.K., and Becker, R.E.: Nurses as psychiatric consultants in a hospital emergency room, Community Mental Health Journal 10:261-267, Fall 1974.
19. Dworkin, A.L., and Dworkin, E.P.: A conceptual overview of selected consultation, American Journal of Community Psychology 3:151-159, June 1975.
20. Mannino, F.V., and Shore, M.F.: Consultation research in mental health and related fields: a critical review of the literature, Public Health Monograph no. 79 PHS 2122, Washington, D.C., 1971, U.S. Government Printing Office.

21. Lippitt and Lippitt, p. 81.
22. Cherniss, C.: The consultation readiness scale: an attempt to improve consultation practice, American Journal of Community Psychology **6**:15-21, February 1978.
23. Jason, L.A., and Ferone, L.: Behavioral versus process consultation interventions in school settings, American Journal of Community Psychology **6**:531-543, December 1978.
24. Mannino, F.V.: Task accomplishment and consultation outcome, Community Mental Health Journal **8**:102-108, May 1972.
25. Reinkind, R.H., Livesay, G., and Kohl, M.: The effects of consultation style on consultee productivity, American Journal of Community Psychology **6**:283-290, June 1978.
26. Stephenson, P.S.: Judging the effectiveness of a consultation program to a community agency, Community Mental Health Journal **9**:253-259, Fall 1973.
27. Watkins, E.L., Holland, T.P., and Ritvo, R.A.: Evaluating the impact of program consultation on health services, Health Education Monographs **3**:385-402, Fall 1975.
28. Woody, R.H.: Process and behavioral consultation, American Journal of Community Psychology **3**:277-285, September 1975.
29. Lippitt and Lippitt, pp. 30-44.
30. Hessler, R.M., New, P.K., and May, J.T.: Power, exchange, and the research-development link, Human Organization **38**:334-339, Winter 1979.
31. Spradley, J.P., and McCurdy, D.W.: Anthropology: the cultural perspective, New York, 1975, John Wiley & Sons, Inc.
32. Breslin, R.W.: Cross-cultural encounters face-to-face interaction, New York, 1981, Pergamon Press.
33. Glaser, W.A.: Experts and counterparts in technical assistance. In Kumar, E., editor: Bonds without bondage: explorations in transcultural interactions, Honolulu, 1979, The University Press of Hawaii.
34. Harvey, R.: Cross-cultural awareness. In Smith, E.C., and Luce, L.F., editors: Toward internationalism: readings in cross-cultural communication, Boston, 1979, Duxbury Press.
35. Morrell, R.: Consultation or control? The cross-cultural advisor-advisee relationship, Psychiatry **35**:264-280, August 1972.
36. Rapoport, R.N.: Some notes on paratechnical factors in cross-cultural consultation, Human Organization **23**:5-10, Spring 1964.
37. Masson, V., International nursing: what is it and who does it? American Journal of Nursing **79**:1244, 1979.
38. Lippitt and Lippitt, p. 1.
39. Bell, C.R. and Nadler, L., editors: The client-consultant handbook, Houston, 1979, Gulf Publishing Co., p. 6.
40. Deloughery and Gebbie, p. 63.
41. Lippitt and Lippitt, pp. 8-26.
42. Lewin, K.: Field theory in social science, New York, 1951, Harper & Row, Publishers.
43. Lippitt and Lippitt, p. 21.
44. Bell, C.R., and Nadler, L.: The client-consultant handbook, Houston, 1979, Gulf Publishing Co., p. 237.
45. Davis, A.J., and Aroskar, M.A.: Ethical dilemmas and nursing practice, New York, 1978, Appleton-Century-Crofts, pp. 1-8.
46. Lippitt and Lippitt, p. 63.
47. Bermant, G., and Warwick, D.P.: The ethics of social intervention: power, freedom, and accountability. In Bermant, G., Kelman, H.C., and Warwick, D.P., editors: The ethics of social intervention, New York, 1978, John Wiley & Sons, Inc., pp. 377-418.

48. Gaup, P.G.: Authority, influence, and control in consultation, Community Mental Health Journal 2:205-210, Fall 1966.
49. Bermant and Warwick, p. 407.
50. Kolter, P.: Marketing for nonprofit organizations, Englewood Cliffs, N.J., 1975, Prentice-Hall, Inc.
51. Montana, P.J.: Marketing in nonprofit organizations, New York, 1978, American Marketing Association.
52. Catalyst staff: Market yourself: the catalyst women's guide to successful resumes and interviews, New York, 1980, G.P. Putnam's Sons.

5

EVALUATION PROCESSES AND TOOLS

Evaluation is an integral part of planning and change. Evaluation provides decision makers with the information needed to make choices. Such information includes the community's needs and wants, how the needs are being addressed, the effects of those efforts, and recommendations for change.

As we noted in Chapter 2, because of the cyclic nature of the planning process, the evaluation phase of one cycle is part of the assessment phase of the next cycle. Even in initial needs assessment for program planning for health and human services, a consultant usually enters a setting in which there are services or programs already seeking to meet some of the needs and wants of the target community and aggregate. Consultants do not start de novo.

Evaluation, as has been the case with every other process we discuss in this book, is a collaborative process. The consultant system, which must include evaluation expertise, interacts with the community system as shown in Fig. 1, p. 16. This interaction takes place in the collaborative intersystem, and this collaborative intersystem becomes a third system, which is made up of components from both consultant and community systems and so is related to each of them but is unique in its own composition and function. Within the collaborative intersystem all of the components of the evaluation process are designed and implemented. It is also here that decisions regarding recommendations for change are developed for use by community suprasystems. For example, in Chapters 7 and 8 we describe two evaluation cases. In each case one or more of us was a member of the consultant system that worked with members of the community system to form the collaborative intersystem in which the evaluations were planned, implemented, evaluated, and reported. The systems in these cases included governmental and community agencies who made use of the findings and implemented the recommendations.

A major reason for conducting any kind of evaluation is to determine what if any changes need to be made in the system studied to bring about a desired outcome. The various components of evaluation (see the box on p. 92) supply decision makers with the data they need to make the best and most objective decisions possible. Thus the feedback from evaluation that indicates the need for change sets the stage for one of two types of system cybernation. The first is cybernation for system regulation. This regulation is accomplished within existing rules and processes. This is the relatively minor kind of fixing we described in Chapter 2 as first-order change. For example, the evaluation shows that a community mental health program is doing a good job meeting the needs specified by its target clientele. A problem that showed up on interviews of a sample of clients and community members is that the program's hours are not convenient for people who work during the day. In discussing the results of the evaluation, the collaborative intersystem recommends that, because limited resources preclude expanding service hours, the program's hours could be changed 2 days a week from 8 AM to 5 PM, as they are now, to 1 PM to 10 PM. If subsequent evaluations indicate that this change in schedule meets the expressed needs of working people, the new schedule will be maintained. If not, further adjustments will be made as indicated.

Some evaluation feedback will necessitate cybernation for system transformation. This is second-order change and requires new approaches, new rules, and systemic change in general. The community mental health collaborative intersystem begins to realize that the population of its target community is changing from middle class, married, working people to less affluent retired people, many of whom, especially the women, are alone. New census data confirm that this is indeed the escalating trend. The collaborative intersystem must change its own membership to include people from the elderly aggregate. After doing so, the reconstituted collaborative group together decides to undertake a needs assessment of the elderly aggregate to guide its planning. This assessment shows, among other things, that many people have impaired mobility, few have their own transportation, many are depressed and lonely, many of the men are not adjusting to retirement and do not know what to do with their time, many of the women have suffered recent significant losses, and many members of the elderly aggregate have serious health needs that are not being adequately treated. The collaborative group realizes that the community mental health center's present staff, facilities, and programs are not appropriate to the needs of this high-risk group. Thus a whole new set of goals and a new plan to achieve them must be developed. Services will have to be taken to the people rather than expecting them to come to the community mental health center. Exchange relationships with agencies that work with elderly people and who have staff with expertise in psychogerontology will have to be developed. Different programs such as grief counseling and recreation facilities will have to be implemented. Much more attention will have to be given to the clients' physical as well as emotional needs. In short, present programs and facilities cannot be fixed; different approaches are needed and must be developed to serve the new changing population.

Not all evaluations result in changes of the magnitude described in the second example. However, community decision makers must be prepared to abandon old programs and ways of doing things to meet changing needs. Such changes are not easy, and people, particularly staff, can get caught in them. Nonetheless, systems must be willing to undertake changes that will transform them and ensure that they remain responsive to the needs of a changing clientele and environment. This is just another example of the reason consultants who collaborate with others in community planning must use caution to avoid the trap of creating services or other programs that are thought to be permanent. As we have said, nothing is permanent except change. To survive, systems need to be ready to undergo second-order as well as first-order change as feedback from evaluations mandate, even though these changes are often difficult.

Patton[1] describes two models on which many program evaluations relied before the 1960s to a greater extent than they do now. The *charity model* focuses on the funders' and the staffs' sincerity and dedication to helping others. Charity model proponents give little priority to scientific evaluation methods. Increasingly, even advocates of this model are coming to realize that, although sincerity and dedication are important components in making a program work, there are alternative courses of action that need to be compared, using more objective guidelines and methods. The plea from communities and aggregates that programs for them are essential must be backed up with qualitative and quantitative evidence that benefits outweigh costs. The shrinking resource base for all kinds of health and human services in the 1980s means that objective evaluations are increasingly important. Programs and services that do not have this kind of evidence of success are less competitive for funds than those that do.

The *pork barrel* model for program evaluation depends on the strength and political influence that the program's constituency wields with decision makers. As we discussed in Chapter 2, collaborative planning involves members of all kinds of groups who will be affected by the program or who have an interest in it. Obviously these groups become the program's constituency from the outset. What happens to the program is of vital and immediate concern to them since they or people close to them are directly involved. The program's continuance is therefore a real issue for its constituency. The more the program's constituency is skillful in terms of politically effective lobbying, the more likely the program is to survive. The block grants for health and social services in the federal budgets of the early 1980s have effectively set the stage at the state level where these monies are allocated for some bitter battles for sufficient funds to ensure that programs continue.

Many consultants have been involved in the intense lobbying efforts that have gone into ensuring that a pet program gets enough money to continue. Those who are most skillful at mobilizing constituents, choreographing testimony, and organizing people to demonstrate, visit, call, or write elected or appointed officials as well as anyone else who is in a position to influence resource allocation decisions are often successful. Even in the absence of objective evaluation data of a program's effectiveness or a community's needs, these kinds of pork barrel approaches often carry weight with both public and private funding agencies. Public agencies are often even more responsive just before election time.

Although the increase of scientific evaluation in the 1970s has reduced reliance on and impacts of the charity and pork barrel models of evaluation, they are by no means extinct. Sound qualitative and quantitative evidence of the effectiveness of a program or the extent of a community's needs derived from well-designed evaluations, when added to the pork barrel and charity approaches, may indeed produce a winning combination. Thus, although the remainder of our discussion of evaluation focuses on more scientific methods for evaluation, we need to remember that the charity and pork barrel approaches still carry political clout. The art is to know when to use each alone or in combination.

EVALUATION COMPONENTS

Components of the evaluation process are presented in the box on p. 92. We have also included some key questions that should be asked at each stage. *Needs assessment* is the initial component in the evaluation process. Needs assessments provide baseline or benchmark information about the current status of the community, aggregate, program, or other system being evaluated. These baseline data form the basis against which comparisons of the outcomes and consequences of subsequent actions will be measured. For example, the needs assessment shows that infant mortality in a community is well above the national average. The collaborative inter-system conducting the evaluations determines that this fact is a priority, since the community wants and needs to reduce its infant mortality. Plans would then be developed to institute efforts to reduce infant mortality in the community. Subsequent stages of the evaluation process would use the baseline data on infant mortality from the needs assessment and evaluation criterion to measure the relative effects of efforts to reduce that rate.

Evaluation of alternative plans of action is the next stage of the evaluation process, after the needs assessment has made clear what should be done. There are two major sets of questions to be answered in this evaluation stage. The first has to do with the consideration of alternative courses of action to bring about desired changes in the situation. Again, in the infant mortality example, alternative plans of action might include improved prenatal services, especially for high-risk mothers; health insurance; increased family planning services, especially for young people, whose risks of both unwanted pregnancy and infant mortality are high; and expansion of food stamp and other nutritional aid programs specifically targeted to women of childbearing age. All of these alternatives involve first-order change. Second-order change alternatives for dealing with infant mortality might include providing all mothers with free comprehensive prenatal, intrapartum, and postpartum services from cer-

EVALUATION COMPONENTS WITH KEY QUESTIONS FOR EACH ONE

NEEDS ASSESSMENT

What is current status?
What does target community need?
What does target community want?

EVALUATION OF ALTERNATIVE PLANS OF ACTION

What are possible alternative actions?
Which one is most likely to yield desired goals?

FORMATIVE EVALUATION

What are clients' experiences?
How well are we progressing toward desired goals?
What changes need to be made to aid that progress?

SUMMATIVE EVALUATION

What was impact on clients?
To what extent did the planned action attain its goals?
What do we do now?

EVALUATION OF COMMUNITY IMPACT

What changes have occurred in community's quality of life as results of the
   program?
What does target community need now?
What does target community want now?

tified nurse midwives and making contraceptive and abortion services available to
anyone desiring them free of charge and with no questions asked. You will recall that
second-order change addresses systemic change and involves the development of
new rules; first-order change functions within existing systems and their rules.

Once the collaborative intersystem has defined the array of alternative actions as
adequately as possible, the second step is to evaluate each one using some set of
objective criteria. These criteria might include cost-benefit analysis, cost-effective-
ness analysis, expert opinion on the most effective alternative based on a review of
the literature, and a survey of the community to see which solutions are most acceptable to the majority.[2] After carefully evaluating all of the alternative actions, the best
solution or a combination of the highest ranking alternatives is chosen and is used as a
basis for planning.

Formative evaluation studies the ongoing process of implementing the chosen
plan of action. If the action is the implementation of a program, the program's
progress toward the desired goals is evaluated at stipulated intervals. Formative
evaluation provides serial answers to several key questions. What are the client's

TABLE 5-1

Comparison of activities in formative and summative program evaluation

Criterion	Formative evaluation	Summative evaluation
Purpose	Ongoing evaluation to increase program's abilities to meet objectives for desired outcomes; gives feedback before and at intervals during conduct of program so that change can be made while program is being implemented	Final evaluation of value of program in terms of attainment of its objectives; provides guidelines for decisions about future of target program(s)
Focus	Processes and their immediate effects vis-a-vis the program's objectives	Outcomes vis-a-vis program's objectives
Process	Prospective or concurrent data gathering and analysis to determine extent to which program is attaining its own objectives as well as other evaluation criteria	Terminal or retrospective summary describing extent to which program has attained its objectives as well as other evaluation criteria
Methods	Uses appropriate design, sampling, and analysis techniques to obtain needed data; prospective and concurrent designs more often used than retrospective designs	Uses appropriate design, sampling, and analysis techniques to obtain needed data; retrospective designs more often used than prospective or concurrent designs
Level of specificity	Very specific to provide guidelines for particular changes in ongoing program	More moderate specificity and more summary in nature to provide guidelines for general decisions about total program
Tone of report	Informal, ad hoc summarization	Formal summarization
Length of report	Varies with findings; as long as needs to be to document needed adjustments	Fairly short to summarize outcomes vis-a-vis objectives and other criteria so that it can be efficiently used by administrators and planners in decision making

Data from Morris, L.L., and Fitz-Gibbon, C.T.: Evaluator's handbook, Beverly Hills, Calif., 1978, Sage Publications, Inc, p. 33.

experiences in the program? This means that evaluators must obtain systematic feedback from clients on their perceptions of services. These data, coupled with information from chart audits, statistical reviews, discussions with staff, and other sources of feedback, are used to address the other pivotal formative evaluation questions: How well are we progressing toward the desired goals? What changes need to be made to aid progress toward goal attainment? Formative evaluations provide the collaborative intersystem group with timely information about the progress of a program. This feedback permits changes to be made during the program's implementation rather than waiting until the end for any systematic evaluation.

Summative evaluation is done at the end of the program. The main questions here are: What impact did the program have on clients? To what extent did the program attain its goals? What do we do now? Client impact is sought by asking clients to evaluate the program in terms of the effects it had on them. Based on client impact data and the comparison of the program's other outcomes with the objectives set for the program at the beginning, the collaborative intersystem group makes recommendations to continue, expand, change, discontinue, or reduce the program. Table 5-1 presents a detailed comparison of formative and summative evaluation activities.

Evaluation of community impact involves longitudinal follow-up after the program or chosen strategy has been implemented for a period of time. The point of evaluating community impact is to answer several questions. What changes have occurred in the community's quality of life since the program that may be related to it? Causation is almost impossible to establish in open social systems because of the tremendous number of interacting variables. Thus evaluations of community impact must infer relationships between the program's activities and changes in the community. To assess changes in a community's quality of life necessitates having criteria that can be used for comparative purposes. Again the needs assessment data that form a baseline of where the community was before planning and programming began is one criterion that can be used in measuring how much change in the indicators has occurred at subsequent times. In Chapter 6 we discuss a number of social indicators and indices that can be used as evaluation tools for assessing community impact.

Other questions that should be addressed in evaluating the impact of programs or other interventions on communities are the same questions that were asked in needs assessment: What does the community want now? What does the community need now? With the asking of these questions, the evaluation process commences again. Thus evaluation, as is planning, is a never-ending cyclic process. We believe that following the evaluation process we have described here, component by component, places into operation the phrase we so often hear regarding evaluation— evaluation is built into the whole program or change process.

EVALUATION PROCESSES

As we shall use them in this discussion, evaluation processes involve the application of research techniques and methods, especially those from the social sciences, to the study of the processes, outcomes, and consequent impacts of plans, programs, and systems on target populations and on communities. Evaluation is similar to research in many ways; it is also different, as Table 5-2 shows. We present the information on research in the table for comparison purposes. Our discussion focuses on evaluation in terms of the criteria in the table.

Purpose

The major purpose of evaluation is to determine to what extent plans and systems are attaining the outcomes and consequences that they were designed to

TABLE 5-2

Comparison of evaluation and research

Criterion	Evaluation	Research
Conduct	Design's purpose is to maximize objectivity of observations; objectives and other criteria on which program, system, or plan is to be judged serve function of hypotheses; often highly eclectic designs to meet needs of specific evaluation	*Experimental:* seeks to control the environment and other variables as much as possible via the research design to test specific hypotheses. *Field:* seeks to describe what is occurring without interference; seeks to generate hypotheses
Instruments	Qualitative and quantitative instruments, many of which are system, program, or plan specific; care should be given to ensure reliability and validity	Qualitative and quantitative instruments, preferably standardized and with established validity and reliability
Confidence limits	Must be congruent with objectives; .10, .20, or .25 may therefore be appropriate[3]	Generally .01 or .05
Use of judgment about value of results	Makes value statement regarding program, system, or plan, i.e., good or bad, successsessful or unsuccessful	Makes no value statement about results
Outcomes	Specific to program(s), system(s), or plan(s) under study; may be subjected via secondary analysis, using general criteria, to enable comparisons with other programs; criteria include cost per unit of service, success/failure ratio, etc.[4]	Generalizable, provided design is sound
Purpose	Assesses systems or plans in terms of attainment of desired outcomes and their consequences; seeks very specific results for use by community decision makers	Develops new knowledge to generate or test hypotheses; seeks generalizable results Applied research that seeks to solve specific problems or meet specific needs for information
Primary audience	Community system and suprasystem; members, e.g., agency administrators, funding agencies, government, and others who must make decisions about changes in or continuation of systems or plans assessed	Scientific and academic communities in pure research, employing agency or industry in applied research, and professional communities
Characteristics of roles	Consultant system serves at pleasure of employing community subsystem and works with community system in collaborative intersystem to plan and to implement evaluation and to develop recommendations; results of evaluation are property of community system or subsystem, not of consultant for such purposes as publication; potential conflicts between consultant and community caused by probable action consequences of evaluation's findings for subsystems, plans, and personnel	Once funding is obtained and study is begun, so long as changes in the protocol are not made, investigator generally has considerable autonomy and few role conflicts; investigator also has considerable control over uses of study's findings in terms of publication and other forms of reporting or replication

Data from Weiss, C.H.: Evaluation research: methods for assessing program effectiveness, Englewood Cliffs, N.J., 1972, Prentice-Hall, Inc., pp. 6-9.

achieve. Under these circumstances, evaluation seeks very specific results that will be of use to the people involved with the plan or system under study. Baseline information on needs and present status of the target aggregate or community described in the initial assessment phase (see box, p. 92) is an important evaluation criterion, since these data provide a basis for measuring change when compared with subsequent data from the same sources. In this context, evaluation is very much like applied research, which also has a specific often problem-oriented focus.

Although most evaluations are quite program specific or system specific, evaluations and other reports from similar programs or systems do form a body of case studies that can be subjected to comparative analyses. Yin and Heald[5] describe the case survey method for analyzing case studies. The instrument is a closed-ended questionnaire or checklist that guides the investigator to report the qualitative and quantitative information in each case study in a reliable, comparable, and aggregative manner. Community planning groups and governing bodies may find this technique useful in helping them to learn from the experiences of others with programs similar to the ones they are considering for development. In so doing, members would develop a list of questions they can ask about each case study obtained from programs similar to the one they are planning. Thus evaluation information may be of use not only to those involved directly with the program but also to others working with similar programs, even though this is not a primary purpose for conducting evaluations.

Primary audience

The community system members who have the responsibility and authority to make decisions about the plan, program, or system are the primary audience for evaluation information about it. These decision makers include planning or governing group members, funding agencies, politicians, and community leaders. Information generated by evaluation processes must be framed in terms that decision makers can use. Recommendations must be specific and operational.

Consultant's roles as evaluator

The consultant system serves at the pleasure of the community system because its overriding point of reference is the community's needs and desired outcomes. Consultants as evaluators in the collaborative intersystem come from inside and outside of the community system to plan and implement evaluation and develop recommendations on the basis of the evaluation findings. Each inside and outside perspective brings strengths and limitations to the collaborative evaluation's efforts for the benefit of the community systems, as seen in Table 5-3.

The results of the evaluation and any reports that evolve are the property of the employing community system and not of the consultant. The community system can decide what to do with the recommendations. The range of decisions is from total

TABLE 5-3

Comparison of selected characteristics of inside and outside evaluator's roles

Criterion	Inside evaluator	Outside evaluator
Credibility	Prophet-in-own-country-syndrome that may reduce credibility	May be viewed as more credible since comes from outside, usually with special credentials and titles
Objectivity	May be "too close to the trees to see the forest;" also may be too personally involved with staff and clients of the program to be able to be objective	May be able to see the forest well but not individual trees; may be able to see more objectively since not personally involved with participants in the program
Access to information	May be given information an outsider cannot hope to get; also may not be able to obtain data that the outsider can	Cannot have the informal contacts an insider does, but may be given access to information that would not be shared with an employee
Competence	Must be competent to carry out the evaluation	Must be competent to carry out the evaluation
Personal investment	May need or want to make things look better than they perhaps are for personal and professional reasons; may be very concerned about what friends and colleagues think of her or his work	Usually more objective and so less likely to make things look better or worse than they are; may be concerned about evaluation by peers in consultation community; also may want to ingratiate self to administrators to ensure subsequent contracts
Breadth of background with similar assignments	Probably limited, although knows this program and agency or community in depth	Usually has substantial experience with similar kinds of program or community evaluations; cannot know program or community to the depth the insider does
Potential for use of results	May have a position in the organization or community with the authority and prestige to influence the use to which recommendations are put	Prestige and authority may motivate agency or community to act on recommendations although outsiders have no formal authority to ensure this
Autonomy	Make take program's or community's assumptions and structures so much for granted as to limit recommendations to first-order changes	May question community's or agency's basic assumptions and structures enough to enable recommendations to include second-order changes if needed
	More likely than an outsider to be fairly closely supervised during evaluation process, which may prove to be an interference; may mean that needed information is more available in some cases and less so in others	More likely than insider to be left fairly unsupervised during process; may mean that access to some needed data is completely missed

Data from Weiss, C.H.: Evaluation research: methods for assessing program effectiveness, Englewood Cliffs, N.J., 1972, Prentice-Hall, Inc., pp. 20-21.

implementation of the recommendations and making public the report to filing the report with no action at all. If the consultant system members want to use the evaluation report or part of the findings for their own purposes, they must obtain permission from the community subsystem to which the report belongs. For us to be able to reprint the report of the Senior Resources Survey in Chapter 8, we had to obtain permission from the Area Agency on Aging, the community subsystem for whom we did the evaluation.

Finally, in terms of roles, consultants must realize that the evaluation process, however collaborative and open it is, is still often perceived as a threat especially to personnel and clients of programs or agencies being evaluated. This is not paranoia but rather a grasp of the reality that evaluations result in recommendations that may mean changes that will affect these people directly. Thus when consultants find that staff and clients are not as cooperative or open as desired, it must be appreciated that the staff and clients have real reasons for their concerns. This anxiety can be reduced if the collaborative intersystem ensures that representatives from these community subsystem groups are well informed, communicate with their constituents, and bring feedback about constituents' concerns back to them. Nonetheless, there will be some resentment and anxiety in almost all evaluations; consultants should not take it personally and should strive to reassure others as much as possible.

As we found in the Senior Resources Survey (see Chapter 8), some agency staff from whom we sought access to volunteer subjects were sufficiently concerned about the possible effects of the survey's findings on their agencies to be very reluctant to cooperate. This reluctance showed up generally in avoidant and obstructionist activities, such as asking us to call back later for a decision, not returning calls, requesting meetings with all of the staff to explain what we were doing and why, cancelling those meetings, and then stalling again on giving us a decision. We were originally tempted to take all of this personally until we realized that the evaluation was perceived as a threat by these staff people. This threat was intensified by the fact that the Area Agency on Aging, with whom we were conducting the evaluation, was the major funding source for many of the agencies we were evaluating, some of whom were the most reticent to cooperate.

Conduct

Patton[6] points out, "Purity of method is no virtue: That strategy is best which matches research methods to the evaluation questions being asked. The challenge is to decide which methods are most appropriate in a given situation." In other words, consultants should design the evaluation study using an eclectic approach to be sure that the methods selected are appropriate for the evaluation at hand. This necessitates that consultants have a broad knowledge of the kinds of designs that are available so that choices may be made from a number of alternative approaches. The overall objectives to follow are to maximize objectivity and to gather the kinds of informtion needed for decision makers to use. We have more to say about designs and evaluation conduct later in this chapter. The program's goals and the system's desired outcomes serve as major evaluation criteria against which findings are judged.

Instruments

The same eclecticism used in deciding how to conduct the evaluation should be used in selecting or developing the instruments. Some of the standardized instruments, such as the *Minnesota Multiphasic Personality Index,* may be appropriate to measure changes in client characteristics as a result of a program's interventions. In many instances the evaluators will have to develop program, community, or aggregate-specific instruments. Reliability and validity testing, in-so-far as feasible, should be done on these specifically developed instruments to be sure that they provide valid and reliable data as a basis for decisions. We discuss a number of kinds of instruments that can be used in evaluations later in the chapter. We are particularly concerned that both quantitative data and qualitative information from clients be sought.

Confidence limits

Confidence limits are a statistical calculation that helps the collaborative evaluation intersystem members and decision makers to see not only whether a program or other activity has made a difference in client or community indicators but also how much change has occurred. As was the case with the selection of design and instrumentation for the evaluation, the confidence limits must also be congruent with the objectives of the program or other activity. This may mean that instead of using .01 or .05 confidence limits, as much quantitative research does, confidence limits of .10 or .20 may be quite rigorous enough for decision making.[3]

Use of judgment about results

The whole purpose of conducting an evaluation is to provide the most reliable, valid, and objective data possible for decision makers to use in deciding on alternative courses of action. Statistics can only tell one whether or not the evaluation's findings are statistically significant; they cannot tell whether the findings are important. The latter is a matter of judgment. To be sure, statistical significance is a useful datum in the decision equation, but in the final analysis, judgment tempered by political, economic, social, and other realities must also be considered in making both recommendations and decisions.

Outcomes

Because of the specificity of the design and instruments to ensure that they are congruent with the objectives of the program or activity being evaluated, the outcomes or findings are generally of value only for making decisions about that program or activity. There are a variety of outcomes of the evaluation process in terms of the kinds of decisions that may be made; some of them follow:

1. Continue the program or activity as it is
2. Terminate the program or activity
3. Expand the program or activity
4. Reduce the program or activity
5. Change the program or activity within the existing system (first-order change)
6. Change the whole program or activity into a new or very different one (second-order change)
7. Develop specific programs or activities for a target community or aggregate
8. Do nothing

ETHICS OF EVALUATION

There are several general ethical issues involved in asking people to participate in evaluations; Babbie[4] gives the following five classifications of ethical issues:

1. Voluntary participation
2. No harm to people being studied
3. Anonymity and confidentiality
4. Researcher's identity
5. Analysis and reporting procedures

His reference is social research and his points are equally applicable for all evaluation components and for all consultants as evaluators.

Voluntary participation

Voluntary participation is a major concern, since subjects have the right to agree or to refuse to participate in evaluations of programs or other activities of which they are a part. We do not refer here to record audit or analysis, but rather to direct personal involvement such as being interviewed or being asked to complete a questionnaire. To decide whether to volunteer or not, people must be told about the evaluation's purpose, how it is being conducted, the risks and benefits likely for them, how their decision will affect their eligibility for other activities or services, and to what use the results will be put. Only then can they give their informed consent to participate.

Guaranteeing people their right to refuse to participate in evaluations in essence means that all of the information that is gathered is obtained from volunteers. This phenomenon introduces probable bias into all evaluations of this type, since people who volunteer to participate may be very different from people who refuse. This probability of bias limits generalizability of the findings to everyone in the program or activity, much less beyond it. This necessity for voluntary participation also essentially eliminates the ability to obtain a truly random sample. Nonetheless, we completely value the principle that people's right to volunteer or to refuse to participate in evaluations outweighs the limitations it brings with it.

No harm to people being studied

No harm to the people being studied means that evaluators must assume responsibility for the protection of people who agree to participate in any kind of research or evaluation. We exclude biomedical research from this discussion, since the risks involved in that type of research are far different from the kinds of social and psychological risks that are involved in the community or program evaluations of interest to us. Just because evaluators are not administering drugs or performing some kind of physical treatment does not mean that evaluations are not without risks to participants. For example, a respondent who is also the client of an agency from which she or he receives services may be at risk of being denied further services if she or he can be identified as giving any kind of negative feedback about the agency. We are loathe to believe that this kind of retaliation can occur, but unfortunately it does. Thus respondents who volunteer to participate in evaluations of services they are receiving must be assured of anonymity for their protection. Often when people are sure that their responses are indeed anonymous, they are more likely to be frank than when their identity can be directly associated with their responses.

In some evaluations, data sought are of a very personal nature and, if made public, could be seriously damaging to respondents. For example, trying to establish a baseline on the extent of substance abuse in a community as a means of justifying the need for drug education, treatment, and rehabilitation programs can place respondents at great risk of arrest if their honest answers can be associated with them. This kind of information is often best gathered by mailed, self-administered questionnaires where respondent anonymity can be safeguarded.

Evaluators must think through the kinds of risks to which evaluations might subject respondents and do the best possible to reduce if not eliminate those risks. Thus the responsibility of risk reduction is a very important consideration in choosing a design and specific methods for the evaluation.

Anonymity and confidentiality

Anonymity and confidentiality are not synonymous, as many people with whom we have worked seem to think. Anonymity means that the evaluator does not know who the respondents are. In the case example in Chapter 7, older persons who volunteered to participate in the assessment were anonymous. The instrument was a self-administered questionnaire on which there were no requests for information that would identify respondents. Respondents were also repeatedly reminded not to put their names or any other personal or individual identifying information on the questionnaires. Those respondents who wished further contact with the evaluators for either counseling or referral services were asked to make their requests separately

CARL A. RUDISILL LIBRARY
LENOIR RHYNE COLLEGE

from the questionnaire, either by approaching the evaluators after completion of the assessment and arranging an appointment or by giving them a note apart from the questionnaire. The evaluators stressed repeatedly to the respondents and to the staff of the agencies in which their respondents were participants that they not only did not need to know personal identity, they did not *want* to know.

Confidentiality means that the evaluators know who the subjects are but do not let anyone else know. Interviews are confidential almost by definition, since the interviewer generally knows the name of the person she or he is interviewing. One must be very careful that this information is kept in a safe place in which others who are unconnected with the evaluation process cannot gain access to it. If an interviewer assures respondents that their identity will not be made known to others, she or he must keep that promise. Such a promise should not be made if the interviewer is not absolutely sure she or he can keep it. If the material one is seeking is at all sensitive, and she or he cannot keep it confidential, the process should be redesigned so that respondents will be anonymous. This alleviates the problem of inadvertent discovery of the identities of respondents in connection with their responses or in any other form.

In the example in Chapter 8, the evaluators were able to separate the respondent's identifying information (i.e., name, address, and phone number), which they had to have to make contact, to describe the study, and, if the person agreed to be interviewed, to make an appointment, from the respondent's answer sheet. The respondent's answer sheet was coded, but this code number did not appear on the respondent's name and address card, which was filed separately and was destroyed at the end of the evaluation. Thus the evaluators were comfortable in assuring these subjects that their identity would be confidential.

Researcher's identity

The researcher's or evaluator's identity must be made known to potential respondents before they are asked to agree to participate in an evaluation. Not only the researcher's name but also the agency or organizational affiliation are important to be sure the respondents understand the program. As shown in the consent form on p. 177 not only was the form on university letterhead, but the names and phone numbers of the evaluators were given. The fact that the evaluation was being conducted by the University of California and the Area Agency on Aging was stated in the first paragraph.

In some evaluations, the evaluator may be tempted to fudge on the exact reasons for the study or for or by whom it is being conducted. Obviously, there are some instances when this kind of deception would be helpful to the quality of the data people are willing to give. If one is conducting a needs assessment for baseline data on the number of substance abusers in a community for the narcotics division of the police department, one is unlikely to get much information if the sponsorship of the assessment is made known to respondents, especially in an interview. Less dramatically, there was a possibility of some reticence on the part of some of the respondents for the Senior Resources Survey to provide feedback on agency services that they needed for fear that they might be denied those services, even though the interviewer assured them this would not be the case.

We believe that the right of potential respondents to know who the evaluator is and for whom the evaluation is being done outweigh the limitations inherent in some instances. The overriding concern again is that the people who agree to participate in evaluations must not come to any harm for doing so.

Analysis and reporting procedures

Analysis and reporting procedures offer another set of ethical issues. The principle of respondent protection again is paramount. Qualitative data should be aggregated, that is, added together and reported in groups. In this way no one person can be identified. In reporting qualitative data one must strike a happy medium between preserving the depth and richness of the material and being sure that respondents cannot be identified preferably even by themselves. Thus names, dates, specific places, and so on must be either deleted or changed. If there is any question, it is better to err on the side of deleting too much rather than too little possible personally identifying information. In the examples in Chapters 7 and 8, we have systematically deleted the names of the specific locales and agencies where the evaluations were done.

Babbie[7] comments on three areas of ethical responsibility that we as evaluators have to our colleagues. All evaluations have some limitations or shortcomings. Some are more important than are others. The point is that readers must be told what the limitations of the evaluation are so that they can judge the evaluation's findings appropriately. For example, in the senior resources survey the convenience nature of much of the respondent sample and the volunteer nature of all of the sample are clearly spelled out.

A major reason for our inclusion of the case examples in Chapters 7 and 8 is to share some of the mistakes we made as well as some of the negative findings we obtained. Too often evaluators are reluctant to report negative results as well as triumphs. The professional community needs to know about both.

Similarly, serendipities, that is, unexpected findings, must be reported as such. Evaluators should not go back to the design and create new hypotheses after the fact to cover serendipitous findings. Rather we should indicate that they are areas for further study. Often these kinds of unexpected findings can prove to be more valuable than the data that were purposely sought.

As a means of pulling many of these ethical considerations together in a readily usable form, we have adapted the Evaluation Subject's Bill of Rights from the "Experimental Bill of Rights" that is used by the University of California, San Francisco.[8]

The Evaluation Subject's Bill of Rights in the box below contains some additional ethical considerations that we will highlight briefly. Subjects should be told about any benefits that they can expect from their participation in the evaluation as well as any risks they may incur. Thus they can do their own cost-benefit analysis before making a decision of whether to participate.

Participants also have the right to refuse to answer any questions and to withdraw from the evaluation at any point. All who have done surveys using self-administered questionnaires have experienced the frustration of receiving questionnaires that are only partially completed. Of course, one can use the data that are there, presuming they are complete, but that does not lessen the dismay over the data that are not provided. Respondents are also free to refuse to answer any question on an interview that they do not want to answer.

The consent form on p. 177 contains the information described in item 7 in the box below. It is very important that respondents be given their own copy to retain should they have any questions after their participation has ended and wish to contact the evaluator for clarification.

In evaluations where an anonymous self-administered questionnaire is used, such as the one in the needs assessment we describe in Chapter 7, the respondents' consent to participate in the study is assumed if they complete any part of the

---

EVALUATION SUBJECT'S BILL OF RIGHTS

1. To be told what the evaluation is trying to find out.
2. To be told what my involvement in the evaluation will be.
3. To be told about any risks that I may experience in particular and how those risks are being minimized.
4. To be told if I can expect any benefit from participating in the evaluation, and if so, what the benefit might be.
5. To be allowed to ask any questions concerning the evaluation both before agreeing to be involved and during the course of the evaluation.
6. To refuse to participate at all or to change my mind about participation in any or all parts of the evaluation at any time after the evaluation is started. My decision about participation will not in any way affect my eligibility for or my experience in any service or activity in this or any other program.
7. To receive a copy of the signed and dated consent form that contains an explanation of the evaluation and how to contact the people in charge.
8. To be free of pressure while considering whether I wish to agree to participate in the evaluation.
9. To be informed of the evaluation's findings, recommendations, and outcomes should I want them.

Modified from Committee on Human Research: Experimental subject's bill of rights. In Guidelines, San Francisco, Calif., 1978, University of California, p. xii.

questionnaire and return it. Since the questionnaire is intended to be anonymous, no identifying information, including a signed consent form, is desired. The introduction to the questionnaire should include the same information that would be on a consent form if one were used: purpose, benefits, risks, content of the evaluation, sponsoring agency, uses to which the information will be put, and the evaluator's name and contact point. This information can be handed out to respondents with the questionnaire if it is administered or included in a cover letter if it is mailed.

Although this is not always the case, it is courteous as well as good personal relations to advise responents how they can obtain a summary of the results of the evaluation if they want them. This offer can be put into operation through the use of an executive summary such as the one completed for the Senior Resources Survey (see p. 239) or through preparing a short news item for the local media. The point is to provide respondents with feedback on the findings of the evaluation. They may be particularly interested in these findings if they have been informed that the findings may influence decisions about programs or other activities that are important to them. Evaluators who are working under contract to conduct evaluations do not have control over the use of the results. The sponsoring agency may not choose to share results with respondents. That is its choice, but evaluators can at least suggest to them that such sharing would be useful to at least some of the respondents.

OVERVIEW OF EVALUATION METHODS

As we have already noted, the objective in selecting designs and instruments to use in evaluations is to match the research methods chosen to the specific evaluation questions asked about a program or other activity. The art is to select the appropriate ones.[9] In this section we discuss a number of research designs, sources of information, and research approaches and instruments that may be of use to you in conducting evaluations. Detailed discussion of analyses and statistical computations is beyond the scope of this book. Here the best we can do is to provide you with à list of resources and to advise you to get consultation from a statistician early. We briefly discuss some of the processes in preparing an evaluation report. Our presentation here is exemplary rather than exhaustive. As a result, we include a number of references that can provide you with far more detail and guidance on all of these areas. This section, as the heading states, is an overview.

Designs

The first consideration in selecting an evaluation design is to formulate the specific questions that the evaluation is to address. If the evaluation is of a program, the questions may focus on the processes or outcomes and how the program's clients perceive these events. This leads us to the second step, which is to decide whether one will use a qualitative or quantitative design to obtain the data to address the evaluation questions. As Patton points out, this decision is "essentially a trade-off between breadth and depth."[10] Using qualitative designs means that the data generated will be rich in detail and description, enabling the evaluator to know a great deal about what the individual respondent believes or thinks about the question she or he is asked. Quantitative design, on the other hand, will provide the evaluator with much more standardized and therefore more easily aggregated and analyzed data. Quantitative designs control respondents much more than qualitative ones do in terms of the amount and kind of information the respondent can give. Let us say that the evaluation question to be addressed is, "How did clients perceive the services they received?" A qualitative approach to gathering data relative to this question could be to use an interview with open-ended questions such as, "Describe your experiences with service X." This approach would enable the client to tell the evaluator in her or his own words what happened to her or him during service X. The interviewer records what the respondent says and may ask probing questions such as "Are there other aspects that you would like to describe? Was this your only experience with service X?" and so forth. The point is to encourage the respondent to continue to describe experiences in her or his own words and from a personal frame of reference until she or he has said everything there is to say.

A quantitative approach to the question of a client's experiences with services might be through the use of a questionnaire in which the respondent is asked to answer a number of questions about the service in terms of the degree to which she or he agrees or disagrees with each statement. This Likert-type scale offers the respondent little opportunity for personal comment and locks her or him into addressing the issues about which the evaluator wants to know. These issues may or may not be those that are most important for the client. A second quantitative approach is to give the client a closed-ended questionnaire, asking for specific knowledge or attitudes or focusing on selected behavioral aspects at the very beginning of the client's participation in the program or service and then at regular intervals throughout. This is an example of a quasi-experimental longitudinal approach to quantitative data. What is sought is change in responses over the time spent in the program, which may or may not be attributable to the client being in the program. We shall define the approaches and designs we have mentioned in this example at greater length. What we want to make clear here is that there is a great deal of difference between qualitative and quantitative approaches to evaluations. Before we do anything more about seeking answers to evaluation questions, evaluators must address the issue of whether we want breadth or depth of information for those questions. Having made this decision, we are ready to move on to the actual design and conduct of the evaluation.

Naturalistic inquiry

Patton describes naturalistic inquiry as research that "does not attempt to manipulate the research setting."[11] This design focuses on qualitative approaches to discovering and describing what is occurring in the setting while changing it as little as possible. As noted in Chapter 1, even observing a situation or phenomenon changes it.[12] Given this, the evaluator tries to introduce little outside influence into the situation being evaluated.

Diesing[13] describes the processes used in naturalistic inquiries. Discovery is the reconstruction of reality via being open to the data that emerge from the setting. Analysis of these data produce the opportunity to verify that data do indeed reflect the reality from which they come. This process leads to what Glaser and Strauss[14] refer to as "grounded theory"; theory that has its basis in inductive and holistic approaches to real phenomena in their own environments.

Some of the approaches and instruments that are useful in naturalistic designs and that we describe briefly later are nonstructured interviews, participant observation, diaries, logs, and critical incidents. Naturalistic inquiry is a major basis for anthropological research.[15]

Case studies

The purpose of case studies is to develop an in-depth description of a single case. The case can be a community system or a specific program. The case study method enables the evaluator to take a comprehensive look at many aspects of the community and to learn from them.[4,16] The richness of detail generated by case studies makes them invaluable aids to planning and evaluation activities. Chapters 7 and 8 contain two case studies of community evaluations. The following texts can be consulted for further examples. Redman[17] provides an excellent example of a case study of the legislative process in his discussion of the development and enactment of the National Health Service Corps. Paul's *Health, Culture, and Community*[18] contains many quoted case studies of community intervention projects.

Although the case study method has many of the advantages of naturalistic studies, so long as evaluators do not manipulate the variables involved, case study designs also have some drawbacks. These include the tremendous time and effort involved in doing them and the difficulties in making comparisons between case studies. Yin and Heald[5] suggest that this shortcoming can be dealt with by using a "case survey method" that in essence subjects cases to analysis by a closed-ended questionnaire to determine whether or to what extent variables are present in the description. Use of this kind of instrument and approach can provide a basis for comparative analysis of a number of case studies on similar communities, programs, or other activities.

Survey

Babbie[19] describes three purposes for survey research. *Description* of the distribution of phenomena or characteristics in a population is the first purpose. For example, the evaluator may be interested in a needs assessment of the number of people in the community who have specific interest in a service. A survey of a sufficiently large random sample of the community's population can give the evaluator an excellent description of the community's need for such a service. *Explanation,* another use for survey research, provides the evaluator with information about why a given phenomenon is distributed in the population as it is. Multivariate analysis, as its name indicates, is a simultaneous examination of two or more variables that can be used to analyze data to produce explanations. For example, data on people's interests may be much more explanatory when analyzed in terms of their age, sex, race, political party, or other independent variables. Much survey research is conducted to learn more about a subject to develop more specific ideas about it and to refine ways of looking at it. This is the *exploratory* use of survey research. All three of these uses of survey research designs are applicable to evaluations.

There are a number of survey research designs. Some of those that are used most frequently in evaluations include cross-sectional designs and longitudinal designs, which use cohorts or panels or study trends.

Cross-sectional designs describe a population at a given point in time. The case examples in Chapters 7 and 8 both used cross-sectional designs. Evaluators need to be cautious in using cross-sectional data for anything more than descriptions, explorations, or explanations of a population's characteristics at the time that the cross-sectional survey is done. Evaluators must beware of trying to predict trends or anything else from a single cross-sectional survey, although these data can be very appropriately used as a baseline against which to compare similar data from subsequent surveys. Thus, cross-sectional surveys are often the design of choice for needs assessments in which the question to be addressed is, "What is the present status of the population in our community regarding the topic in which we are interested?"

Longitudinal survey designs are used to provide descriptive, exploratory, or explanatory data on a population over a period of time. In other words, they are serial cross-sectional surveys. Trend surveys look at changes over time. The serial Gallup polls before elections are an example of trend surveys. These polls show the changes in people's attitudes toward candidates or issues on the ballot.

Panel surveys focus on a group of responents over time, such as evaluations that periodically survey the same sample of agency clients over time to describe and explain the changes in their attitudes, behaviors, or other characteristics. Panel surveys are useful informative evaluations because they provide information from the same group of clients during the life of the program. Results of these panel surveys provide decision makers with information that can help them in deciding what, if any, changes are needed in the program.

Cohort surveys are periodical surveys of samples of a population that have some common characteristic. A faculty decides that it will conduct a cohort survey of its graduates every 3 years to determine whether they are working and the kinds of positions they hold and to invite feedback to help the faculty adjust the curriculum.

Thus in 1983 a sample of graduates from 1980 would be drawn and sent the survey instrument. In 1986 another sample of the graduating class of 1980 would be surveyed in a similar manner.

Although both panel and cohort surveys sample people from the same group, panel surveys use the same sample of respondents over time and cohort surveys use different samples entirely. As long as the evaluator has access to an accurate list of the total population group from whom to sample, so that everyone in the group has an equal chance of being selected for the survey at each stipulated interval, the condition for a random sample for a cohort study is met. Panel studies are drawn randomly once and then this same sample is used throughout the subsequent stages of the longitudinal survey design. Many evaluators and researchers have written about survey methods.[4,20-23]

Quasi-experimental designs

We will now discuss the designs in which the evaluator consciously and systematically manipulates one or more variables to see what the effects are on other phenomena. The variables the evaluator manipulates are called the independent variables. The variables that are thought to be responsive to those manipulations are the dependent variables. In true experimentation, the evaluator would be able to control and manipulate the independent variables to a considerable extent. Other characteristics of experimental design are the use of a control or a comparison group and a treatment or a study group. Subjects in the experiment are assigned randomly to each of the study and control groups. Since it is usually not possible to meet these conditions in community and organizational evaluations because of the evaluator's inability to control groups or to have a comparable control group at all, one is generally only able to conduct quasi-experimental evaluations rather than truly experimental ones.

For example, the following is a common quasi-experimental evaluation design. A group of people are offered a class on some component of health promotion. At the outset of the class, the participants are given a test to establish their baseline knowledge of the subject to be covered in the class. At the end of the class, they are given exactly the same test. A comparison of the before and after scores is used as an evaluation of the extent to which the class has learned the material. Assuming that the questions asked on the pretest and posttest were related to the material taught in between and that the respondents' scores were higher on the posttest than on the pretest, it can be inferred that the respondents learned something from the class. In this example, the evaluator controlled the independent variable, the class, and measured the effects of the independent variable, the class, on the dependent variable, respondent learning. This is a very simple illustration. It can be made more complex and more rigorous in the process by such procedures as random assignment of learners to the class and to another kind of program that has nothing to do with the material being taught in the class. The same pretest and posttest procedure is conducted on both groups. The differences in the pretest and posttest scores of the control group, that is, those who did not have the health promotion class but rather only the pretest and posttest for the health promotion class, are a reflection of the effect of the learning that took place by simply doing the pretest. Again, this is a simple example. Quasi-experimental designs are potentially much more complex and we suggest additional reading to guide your use of these very appropriate approaches to evaluations.[24-26]

Sources of data

As with the selection of evaluation designs, the choice of sources of data for the evaluation must be dictated by the questions the evaluation seeks to have answered. For example, if the evaluation focuses on the effects on clients of group therapy, then clients must be a major source of information. Other sources may be used to supplement client responses and evaluations, but they cannot substitute for them.

The following list is a selection of possible data sources. Reading through it may suggest still others to you that you may wish to use instead of or in addition to some of these.

1. Client responses
2. Client records
3. Agency or organization records and other documents
4. Observations by staff or others
5. Staff and administration responses
6. Secondary sources such as reports from other people, books, newspaper articles, and data from other agencies
7. Surrogate or substitute sources
8. Social indicators

Within limits of time and other resources for the conduct of evaluation, the more appropriate sources of data the evaluator can use to provide information to answer the evaluation questions, the more likely the evaluation will provide valid and reliable answers to those questions.

DATA-GATHERING APPROACHES

Before presenting some of the more commonly used data-gathering approaches for evaluations, we need to briefly raise a few overriding considerations. Validity, the ability of an approach to measure what it is intended to measure, is a concern evaluators must address when developing instruments that are specific to their own programs. Pretesting with people who are similar to those who will actually use the instrument is one way to increase its validity, as is having people from the agency or community system who really know what it is to be evaluated collaborate in the development of the instrument.

Reliability has to do with consistency or the ability of the instrument to repeatedly measure the same phenomenon. Reliability addresses the instrument's appropriateness for use in a given situation. For example, an instrument developed to evaluate child-care centers will probably not be reliable for use in evaluating outpatient clinics.

No matter how well developed the instrument is in terms of reliability and validity if the directions given to the respondents who have agreed to participate in the evaluation are not clear, the data obtained may be useless. Therefore, in addition to pretesting the items on the questionnaire or other instrument, the evaluator must also pretest the instructions that will be used. Changes suggested by the pretesters should be made and the instructions should be pretested again. Clear unambiguous directions are essential on all evaluation instruments, but none more so than on mailed questionnaires with which respondents cannot ask questions.

Finally, one must make sure that the language used in the evaluation instrument is understandable to the people who will be participating. If a number of program clients speak a language other than English, the instrument should be translated into their language and carefully pretested to be sure that the translation is both linguistically and conceptually accurate. It must be remembered that not everyone reads well and some respondents may have trouble comprehending what the evaluator thinks is perfectly clear language. Others, especially the elderly, may have impaired sight. The consent form for the Senior Resources Survey in Chapter 8 is in large type to be sure that respondents can see the words. Careful and repeated pretesting of the instrument before its use can help evaluators to deal with these and many other instrument problems. We cannot stress strongly enough the need for pretesting.

Sample selection is another area in which process is terribly important. The sample of choice in most studies is a random one. In random sampling every participant in a program has an equal chance of being selected. This requires a complete and accurate listing or some other vehicle to facilitate random choosing. Either a table of random numbers or the toss of a die can be used to start the sampling process. The following references can assist you in random and other kinds of sampling processes. [4,20,23,27]

Table 5-4 describes some of the major advantages and disadvantages of a number of instruments and qualitative approaches used in evaluations. Next to the data-gathering approach are references that you may wish to consult for more information about the approach.

ANALYSIS OF EVALUATION RESULTS

The importance and complexity of data tabulation and analyses make their adequate discussion beyond the scope of this book. Many community agencies and planning bodies have statisticians on their staffs. Evaluators would be well advised to become acquainted with people who have these skills early in the evaluation process.

TABLE 5-4

Advantages and disadvantages of selected data-gathering approaches that may be used in evaluations

Data-gathering approaches	Advantages	Disadvantages
Participant observations[15,28]	Yield verbal and nonverbal data Promote access to privileged and detailed information because of high degree of evaluator involvement in the setting Involve minimal evaluator manipulation and control of variables Allow for flexible use of a variety of techniques	May be problematic for evaluator entry and acceptance in population Require great skill and interpersonal sensitivity Involve tremendous amount of time Require considerable evaluator adaptation to the setting Make analysis and interpretation of data difficult Alter situation by observer's presence
Face-to-face unstructured interviews[29,30]	Provide in-depth information Enable discussion of sensitive topics, assuming development of evaluator rapport Allow observation of nonverbal responses	Very expensive May embarrass respondent and result in termination of the interview if sensitive topics are broached Require careful interviewer preparation May intensify variation in reliability within and among raters
Face-to-face structured interviews[29-31]	Allow observation of nonverbal responses More easily analyzed than open-ended interviews Permit less variation of reliability within and among raters than open-ended interviews	Prevent spontaneous interchange Very expensive
Performance appraisals of client behavior[32]	More reliable than reports of performance Provide assessments in real rather than contrived situation	Alter situation by observer's presence Require observer time on a one-to-one basis, therefore expensive May intensify variation of reliability within and among raters
Telephone interviews[20,22]	Provide in-depth information Reduce embarrassment of discussing sensitive topics face to face Conserve interviewer's time Do not involve travel and energy use	Expensive, especially if using long-distance calls Bias sample to those who have phone service Provide no observation of nonverbal responses Require careful interviewer preparation

Method	Advantages	Disadvantages
Logs, diaries, and critical incidents[33-35]	Provide rich qualitative data on personal experiences Less expensive than direct observation	Difficult to analyze Very time consuming and may result in incomplete information
Administered questionnaires*	Relatively easy to complete and tabulate with closed-ended items Provide rich data with open-ended items Relatively nonthreatening when gathering sensitive information Provide opportunity for respondents to clarify directions and items by asking evaluator Able to reach large sample	Require literacy Difficult to analyze with open-ended items Limit data respondents can give with closed-ended items May compromise reliability by evaluator's answers to questions
Self-administered mailed questionnaires*	Relatively easy to complete and tabulate with closed-ended items Provide rich data with open-ended items Relatively inexpensive to administer even with round-trip postage Nonthreatening when gathering sensitive information Able to reach large sample	Require literacy Difficult to analyze with open-ended items Must provide directions and items that are clear and unambiguous since there is no way for respondents to ask questions Limit data respondents can give with closed-ended items Present difficulty in following up incomplete or nonresponses
Semantic differentials[36-38]	Relatively easy to complete, assuming respondent understands dicotomous variables and continuums Easily tabulated and analyzed Can be treated as interval data	Limit data respondents can give with closed-ended items May have response-set bias
Likert scales[39,40]	Easily tabulated and analyzed Can be treated as interval data Relatively easy to complete, assuming respondent understands intervals and continuums	Limit data respondents can give with close-ended items May allow respondents to check more than one category May have response-set bias
Paper-and-pencil evaluations of clients	May employ standardized instruments if appropriate to evaluation objectives Relatively inexpensive to administer and score if closed-ended items are used	Difficult to analyze with open-ended items May not have available standardized instruments that are appropriate to evaluation objectives May not be able to construct valid or reliable program-specific ad-hoc instruments

Continued.

Modified from How to evaluate health programs, vol. 1, Washington, D.C., 1978, Capitol Publications, pp. 1-6.
*References 4, 6, 20, 22, 29.

TABLE 5-4

Advantages and disadvantages of selected data-gathering approaches that may be used in evaluations—cont'd

Data-gathering approaches	Advantages	Disadvantages
Rating scales[41]	Easily completed Can provide relatively objective data, assuming respondent understands categories	May intensify variation in reliability within and among raters Limit data respondent can give with closed-ended items May have response-set bias
Ranking scales[41]	Can provide relatively objective data, assuming respondent understands categories Easily analyzed	Difficult for many respondents to understand Hard to rank many variables Limit data respondent can give with closed-ended items
Q-sorts[42,43]	Force respondents to make choices Reduce response-set bias	Require literacy Require understanding of procedure and clear directions Time consuming Limit data respondents can give with forced choices
Record reviews (chart audits)[44]	Do not involve subject directly Unobtrusive Do not require special skills for data gathering Relatively inexpensive Relatively reliable as long as record format does not change and data are appropriately recorded	Limited to available data Often difficult to validate May not always completely provide data desired

They should be drawn into the collaborative intersystem, since their consultation on the development and even the way an instrument is set up on paper can greatly influence the ease with which the data can be handled. As we said in the introduction of this chapter, find help from a statistician early. The following references will be of help to you with or without a statistician.*

REPORTING EVALUATION RESULTS

The purpose of presenting a report of the evaluation is to let people know what you did, what you found, and the recommendations the findings suggest. Our report of the Senior Resources Survey in Chapter 8 follows a fairly standard format[53,54]:

1. Background to introduce the setting and agencies involved in the evaluation
2. Purpose or why the evaluation was undertaken
3. Methods used in the evaluation; all instruments and other forms connected with the evaluation should be appended to it
4. Limitations of the evaluation so that the reader is aware of these before reading the results and can weigh the results in light of the reported limitations
5. Findings and analyses in as clearly usable a form as possible

The collaborative intersystem that was responsible for this evaluation decided that the findings of the survey should be presented as clearly as possible with a minimum combining of information. Thus there are many more tables in this report than many of you will choose to put in your own.

The best rule of thumb that we know to use as a guide on how to prepare the report is to work closely with the people and agencies who will use it. Together you can develop a report that will fairly present the data the evaluation generated and be in a usable form for the people who will need it for planning or other purposes.

SUMMARY

We have used this presentation on evaluation to discuss five evaluation components (needs assessment, evaluation of alternative plans of action, formative evaluations, summative evaluations, and evaluation of community impact), evaluation processes, and an overview of evaluation methods. In the section on ethics in evaluation, we dealt with informed consent and presented an evaluation subject's Bill of Rights.

*References 21, 22, 24, 35, 45-52.

REFERENCES

1. Patton, M.Q.: Utilization-focused evaluations, Beverly Hills, Calif., 1978, Sage Publications, Inc.
2. Thompson, M.S.: Benefit-cost analysis for program evaluation, Beverly Hills, Calif., 1980, Sage Publications, Inc.
3. Morris, L.L., and Fitz-Gibbon, C.T.: Evaluator's handbook, Beverly Hills, Calif., 1978, Sage Publications, Inc., p. 33.
4. Babbie, E.R.: The practice of social research, ed. 2, Belmont, Calif., 1979, Wadsworth Publishing Co., Inc.
5. Yin, R.K., and Heald, K.A.: Using case survey method to analyze policy studies, Administration Science Quarterly **20:**371-381, September 1975.
6. Patton, M.Q.: Qualitative evaluation methods, Beverly Hills, Calif., 1980, Sage Publications, Inc., p. 17.
7. Babbie, p. 64.
8. Committee on Human Research: Experimental Subject's Bill of Rights. In Guidelines, San Francisco, 1978, University of California, p. xii.
9. Patton, 1980, p. 17.
10. Patton, 1980, p. 97.
11. Patton, 1980, p. 41.
12. Flynn, P.A.: Holistic health: the art and science of care, Bowie, Md., 1980, Robert J. Brady Co., pp. 1-4.
13. Diesing, P.: Patterns of discovery in social sciences, Chicago, 1971, Aldine Publishing Co., p. 15.
14. Glaser, B.G., and Strauss, A.L.: Discovery of grounded theory: strategies for qualitative research, Chicago, 1967, Aldine Publishing Co.
15. Pelto, P.J., and Pelto, G.H.: Anthropological research: the structure of inquiry, ed. 2, Cambridge, Mass., 1978, Cambridge University Press.
16. Pelto and Pelto, pp. 235-243.
17. Redman, E.: The dance of legislation, New York, 1973, Simon & Schuster, Inc.
18. Paul, B.D., editor: Health, culture, and community: case studies of public reactions to health programs, New York, 1955, Russel Sage Foundation.
19. Babbie, E.R.: Survey research methods, Belmont, Calif., 1973, Wadsworth Publishing Co., Inc., pp. 58-59.
20. Dillman, D.A.: Mail and telephone surveys: the total design method, New York, 1978, John Wiley & Sons, Inc.
21. Polit, D., and Hungler, B.: Nursing research: principles and methods, New York, 1978, J.B. Lippincott Co., pp. 195-208.
22. Simon, J.L.: Basic research methods in social sciences: the art of empirical investigation, ed. 2, New York, 1978, Random House, Inc.
23. Weisberg, H.F., and Bowen, B.D.: An introduction to survey research and data analysis, San Francisco, 1977, W.H. Freeman and Co., Publishers.
24. Cook, T.D., and Campbell, D.T.: Quasi-experimentation: design and analysis issues for field settings, Chicago, 1979, Rand McNally & Co.
25. Polit and Hungler, pp. 147-174.
26. Campbell, D.T., and Stanley, J.C.: Experimental and quasi-experimental designs for research, Chicago, 1963, Rand McNally & Co.
27. Babbie, 1979, pp. 159-200.
28. McCall, G.J., and Simmons, J.L.: Issues in participant observation: a text and reader, Menlo Park, Calif., 1969, Addison-Wesley Publishing Co., Inc.

29. Polit and Hungler, pp. 325-356.
30. Patton, 1980, pp. 121-265.
31. Payne, S.L.: The art of asking questions, Princeton, N.J., 1951, Princeton University Press.
32. Webb, E.J., and others: Unobtrusive measures: nonreactive research in the social sciences, Chicago, 1966, Rand McNally & Co.
33. Simon, pp. 194, 296.
34. Polit and Hungler, pp. 230-233.
35. Waltz, C., and Bausell, R.B.: Nursing research: design, statistics, and computer analysis, Philadelphia, 1981, F.A. Davis Co.
36. Polit and Hungler, pp. 366-368.
37. Simon, pp. 410-411.
38. Weisberg and Bowen, pp. 50-51.
39. Babbie, 1979, pp. 409-420.
40. Polit and Hungler, pp. 361-364.
41. Waltz and Bausell, pp. 94-97.
42. Waltz and Bausell, pp. 93-94.
43. Polit and Hungler, pp. 391-393.
44. Webb and others, pp. 53-111.
45. Weisberg and Bowen, pp. 96-225.
46. Rosenberg, M.: The logic of survey analysis, New York, 1968, Basic Books, Inc., Publishers.
47. Rossi, C.H., and Freeman, H.E.: Evaluation: a systematic approach, Beverly Hills, Calif., 1982, Sage Publications, Inc.
48. Cohen, J.: Statistical process analysis for the behavioral sciences, rev. ed., New York, 1977, Academic Press, Inc.
49. Dever, G.E.A.: Community health analysis: a holistic approach, Germantown, Md., 1980, Aspen Systems Corp.
50. Huff, D.: How to lie with statistics, New York, 1954, W.W. Norton & Co., Inc.
51. Davis, J.A.: Elementary survey analysis, Englewood Cliffs, N.J., 1971, Prentice-Hall, Inc.
52. Fitz-Gibbon, C.T., and Morris, L.L.: How to calculate statistics, Beverly Hills, Calif., 1978, Sage Publications, Inc.
53. Morris, L.L., and Fitz-Gibbon, C.T.: How to present an evaluation report, Beverly Hills, Calif., 1978, Sage Publications, Inc.
54. Weisberg and Bowen, pp. 222-229.

6

SOCIAL INDICATORS

As we have throughout the book, in this presentation of social indicators and social indices, we stress the need for those who work in collaborative systems with members of communities to have the best possible data on which to base and evaluate plans and activities. Because of their importance throughout the work of consultants with others, social indicators along with holism and systems theory provide consultants with a conceptual and informational framework (see Fig. A in the preface).

The entire field of social indicators is complex and rather controversial. Notwithstanding this reality, never before have reliable, valid, and current social indicator data been more important for planning and evaluating changes in communities than they are now. At the time that this book is being written, federal, state, and local budgets for health and human services are being drastically cut. These cuts threaten many vital direct client services; they also have the potential to curtail the collection, analysis, and dissemination of many of the kinds of social indicator data discussed in this chapter. One way to be sure that the real outcome and long-term effects of health and human services budget cuts cannot be clearly measured by any agency or interested party is to dismantle the reporting system that has the capacity to quantify and report such impacts. Despite this unhappy political reality, consultants continue to need the best possible social indicator data to use in work with communities. In this chapter we briefly discuss the background and development of the social indicators movement and social indicators. We stress the essential requirement that all social indicators that are used in working collaboratively with the members of a community must be based in theory and must be congruent with the conceptual framework and objectives of the changes they seek to bring about. We present several definitions and a number of characteristics of social indicators and indices. We describe a systems model of a community planning and evaluation process that uses social indicators and indices as major input into the process and changes in these measurements as major consequences of its outcomes. The chapter concludes with the Physical Quality of Life Index as an example.

HISTORY OF SOCIAL STATISTICS AND SOCIAL INDICATORS

The word *statistics* is derived from the Latin *statisticus*, pertaining to a statist or one who believes in the sovereignty of the state.[1] The first modern recorded census was done in Quebec in 1665. In 1690 Sir William Petty in England published his *Political Mathematics*, which he saw as a means to describe the state and to assess taxes.[2,3,4] In 1928 Lambert Quetelet, a Belgian, published a statistical handbook on his country that is credited with being the first modern attempt at social quantification.[5] In the twentieth century (in 1924), A.C. Pigou,[6] a British economist, in his *The Economics of Welfare,* urged consideration of social costs that had largely been ignored in the development of capitalism and the Industrial Revolution.

In the United States, at the University of Chicago, William Ogburn became director of research for the Research Committee on Social Trends that President Hoover created in 1929 and so was able to pursue his interest in developing theory and improved measurement of social change. The advent of the Great Depression and the Second World War turned governmental attention to economic indicators and away from studies of social trends until the 1960s.[7]

The Kennedy administration revived interest in social-trend analysis, in contrast to the emphasis on econometric data and cross-sectional social data that had predominated in the United States for the previous 20 or more years. The American Academy of Arts and Sciences was commissioned to undertake a project to assess the nature and extent of unintended consequences of the United States space program.[8] Raymond Brauer[9] edited the Academy's landmark report in 1966. Brauer is credited with being the father of the social indicators movement.[8] At the same time, the Russell Sage Foundation became interested in social indicators and chose to focus its work on theoretical concerns.[10,11,12] The term *social indicator movement* was coined by Otis Dudley Duncan[13] in 1969. The United States government has published a series of reports entitled *Social Indicators*, the first in 1973, then in 1976, and the most recent one in 1980. The National Center for Health Statistics, which is discussed later, also provides a wealth of health-related materials. United States government publications can be obtained from the U.S. Government Printing Office. The Bureau of the Census has had a Social Indicators Office since 1977.[14]

On an international level, the Organization for Economic Cooperation and Development (OECD) has undertaken a massive social indicators development program.[15,16] The United Nations has developed a system of social and demographic statistics. In addition, the United Nations and the World Health Organization are much involved in the social indicators movement.[17,18] A complete review of the kinds of efforts being undertaken by all of these agencies as part of the social indicator movement is obviously beyond the scope of this book. Our aim here is to introduce the subject and to provide those of you who are interested in reading more about the activities of these and other agencies with an introduction to the resources available.

Statistics and their progeny, social indicators, have grown up in an atmosphere of some conflict. Some have seen them as a means to measure individual and social well-being as well as changes in the status of these measurements. Others have seen and perhaps still see statistics and social indicators as instruments for planning and thereby as a means for social control.[3] In Chapter 2 we spoke about the attitudes toward planning that vary from desires for considerable control to the belief that there should be no interference with the course of events. How members of any collaborative intersystem view statistics and social indicators and how they choose to use them has much of its roots in their attitudes toward the appropriateness of various levels of social control and manipulation. This is a major philosophical issue that each human service worker must address personally as a consultant, planner, evaluator, or whatever other collaborative role she or he plays. Human service workers need to facilitate their counterparts' deliberations on the issue as well. We believe that social data are essential for rational planned change in systems as well as serving as a basis for evaluations of the outcomes and consequences of those change activities. Again we stress our overriding commitment to full collaboration in all parts of the planning process by the people who will be affected by the changes that are made.

There are many other sources of information on social indicators. *Social Indicators Research* contains articles of the development and use of social indicators. Most journals in the social and health fields periodically have articles on social indicators.

FRAMEWORK FOR USE OF SOCIAL INDICATORS
Conceptualizations

Before we discuss some of the definitions and characteristics of social indicators, we begin by stressing that the social indicators used in the work of consultants must be grounded in some rational way with theories and concepts that have some scientific validity and acceptance. The lack of this kind of conceptual validity has been a problem with much of the development and use of social indicators to date.[19] This problem has been compounded by several factors. Systematically and comparably collected data in many geographical areas and on a number of phenomena are lacking. For example, the United States Census provides a great deal of data about selected phenomena for standard metropolitan statistical areas (SMSAs), those geographical areas with 50,000 or more people, but very little information on less densely populated areas.[20] For those who work with urban communities that qualify as standard metropolitan statistical areas there is a veritable feast; for those who work in rural communities there is much more of a famine. Much of the social indicator development in the past has been on a more or less ad hoc basis to address immediate policy needs; much of the data used for these purposes have been both atheoretical and unsystematically developed.[4] Also the quality of the conceptual basis for social indicators is highly dependent on the ongoing development and testing of social theory in general. The more valid and reliable are our social theories, the more valid and reliable will be our measurements of their prevalence and effects. De Neufville[2] gives a beautiful example of the status of much of social science as a basis for the development of social indicators:

> Efforts have gone on for at least 75 years to define and measure poverty. The real obstacle is clearly the conceptual one rather than the technical one. The very basic decision has not been made whether poverty is a level of material well-being, a relative condition, or a state of mind. Even if that is decided, the concept is still too general to measure.

Carlisle[22] speaks of social indicators as "operational definitions" of concepts that describe a social system. This means that one must have some knowledge of the social concepts that are relevant to the collaborative activities for community change in which one participates. This conceptual grounding for data generation and use is a contribution that a consultant, planner, or evaluator can make. Rossi and Gilmartin[23] provide some help:

> The best way to ensure that a concept is appropriately designed for use in developing social indicators is to narrow down its definition using the hypothesized relations among the relevant variables in the theoretical framework.

They give the example of the socioeconomic status (SES) that has been variously defined in terms of father's occupation, family income, type and ownership of dwelling, and a variety of other variables.[23] The way to select an appropriate variable or variables for a concept such as socioeconomic status is to choose those that are congruent with the theoretical framework of the assessment, evaluation, planning, or other activity. Say that one is working with a community-based program group to determine a reasonable user fee for its program. The objectives include developing an equitable scale of payment rather than a regressive one. The operational definition of socioeconomic status one might choose to use in this instance could be based on total family income and the amount of income remaining after fixed expenses such as rent or mortgage payments, food, auto or other installment payments, medical care, and other regular budget items have been paid. This operational definition might not be applicable to other program-participant socioeconomic status evaluations; they would have to develop their own operational definitions of the concepts they are using. The point here is that whatever social indicators one chooses to use, they must be consciously based in theory, and the concepts must be as clearly operationally defined as possible.

Definitions

There are a number of definitions of social indicators; the number reflects both the field's relative infancy and the controversies in it. Land[24] offers a general definition with which we will begin our discussion:

Social indicators are statistics which measure social condition and changes therein over time for various segments of a population. By social conditions, we mean both the external (social and physical) and the internal (subjective and perceptual) contexts of human existence in a given society.

We have already noted that statistics are a tool that is used to describe the state; in our discussion we will focus primarily on statistics that describe the community with which one is working. There are many kinds of statistics; six were identified by the Conference of European Statisticians[25]:

1. *Raw statistical series* such as the data presented in the United States Census. These data are simply presented without discussion, elaboration, or interpretation.
2. *Key statistical series,* such as those found in the United States Census, present an array of selected statistics that are all thought to be related to social conditions.
3. *Comprehensive systems of statistics* are found in the United Nations' system of social and demographic statistics.
4. *Composite indices* are illustrated by the Physical Quality of Life Index, which we will discuss later.
5. *Synthetic representative series* are computed by the use of statistical techniques such as multivariate analysis, multiple regression, and discriminant analysis. (See the reference section of Chapter 5 for sources of information on these techniques.)
6. *Series that fit into social models* are labeled as such because they are designed to specifically address the concepts of the social models they are intended to describe.

Carley[26] argues that all approaches to social data except *raw statistical series* should be considered to be social indicators, since this is indeed what is being done and since these five approaches to social data are all useful for policy decisions. The use of social indicators as policymaking tools has been a major factor in their development.

Carlisle[22] describes four uses of social indicators in the policy-making process:

1. *Information indicators* that are descriptive of the society and changes that are occurring. These kinds of indicators could include serial data on population mobility and changes in crime rates, unemployment, or other phenomena over time. Again, these indicators describe but do not seek to analyze or explain the changes they show.
2. *Predictive indicators* based on social theory. Their presence in a community is viewed conceptually as predictive of the development or presence of related phenomena. For example, population density is an indicator of crowding that is thought to be related to poverty, high crime rates, and other symptoms of social pathology. We would prefer to call these kinds of indicators warning or symptomatic indicators rather than predictive ones, since

social phenomena have multiple causations. Careful analysis is required to determine whether indicators such as high population density are even related to other phenomena such as crime. If they are related, further study is needed to ascertain whether the relationship is merely correlational or if it is indeed part of multiple causation.

3. *Problem-oriented indicators* are normative based in that to define a problem, one must have a conceptualization of what is "good" and what is "bad," since problems are generally thought to be "bad" and so need to be fixed. Problem-oriented indicators are those that precipitate the development of policies and of their resultant programs to promote such behaviors as use of prenatal care or to reduce others such as juvenile crime.

4. *Program evaluation indicators* are those data sources that are used to monitor the effects, both outcomes and consequences, of policies and programs. As we discussed in Chapter 5, evaluation criteria are operationalizations of program objectives and the effectiveness of a program is judged, at least in part, in terms of its level of attainment of those objectives.

All of these types of indicators are valued for their utilitarian applications to a community's needs.

Murnaghan[27] defines health indicators as "statistics selected from the larger pool because they have the power to summarize, to represent a larger body of statistics, or to serve as indirect proxy measures for information that is lacking." Certainly the characteristics she specifies are as important to all kinds of social indicators as they are to health indicators. Let us look at them individually.

Anyone who has worked with the masses of data that are available from and about most communities has at times felt that she or he was overwhelmed. There are literally thousands of bits and pieces of information that can be or have been generated. Some kind of shorthand or summary is desperately needed. The social indicator, socioeconomic status, that we have already mentioned, is an example of such an attempt at shorthand or summary presentation of data relating to a complex concept. The infant mortality rate has long been used throughout the less developed world as a shorthand way of looking at or indicating the status of health care, sanitation, and other social and environmental conditions.[27-29] Again we stress that regardless of what indicator is chosen to describe the target community or population, it must be firmly rooted in a conceptual framework.

Murnaghan's definition of health indicators introduces an important aspect of the whole field—the idea of indicators as proxies, substitutes, or surrogates for phenomena that are hard to measure directly. Health is an excellent example of a concept that defies direct measurement. Part of the problem is caused by an inadequate conceptualization of what health is that makes its operationalization and subsequent measurement not only very difficult, but also potentially invalid and unreliable. A surrogate measurement that one of us has used elsewhere is *optimal level of functioning* (OLOF).[30] The conceptual basis for this surrogate measurement or indicator of health is that people's own definition of and level of satisfaction with their ability to do what they want with their lives is a more valid indicator of health than are such measures as a physician's certification of a disease-free state or absence of hospitalization or disability. Optimal level of functioning brings one back to Land's concerns for measuring "internal (subjective and perceptual) contexts of human existence."[31] We shall have more to say about subjective and objective indicators shortly. In the meantime, we must stress that even greater consideration of the conceptual basis of proxy or surrogate indicators is needed than is the case for direct indicators.

Snider[32] identifies four categories of social statistics that are useful in producing social indicators. They are applicable to our focus on work with communities or aggregates.

1. *Objective or factual information* includes incidence and prevalence rates for various conditions in a population group or clients' answers on a pre- and post-test.
2. *Subjective or attitudinal data* include client satisfaction surveys in which a program's clients are asked to evaluate services they have received. These kinds of data are also referred to as qualitative data.[33] We view them as an essential component of any community activity that involves people.
3. *Behavioral or user information* such as observations of clients' activities might include noting improved skills in a recreational activity or activities of daily living. User information focuses on the number of agencies clients have used.
4. *Demographic and social background variables* include age, sex, income, and racial distributions in a population or the number of owner-occupied dwellings. These are kinds of data that the United States Census and the periodically issued *Social Indicators* present.[34]

These definitions point out different types of and uses for social indicators according to a number of authors and groups. For our purposes, we shall use social indicators as conceptually based data that measure social conditions and can be used for comparative purposes within and among communities and for policy making. Having derived this definition, we now turn to address selected characteristics of social indicators.

CHARACTERISTICS OF SOCIAL INDICATORS

Rossi and Gilmartin[35] present a number of characteristics of social indicators that can serve as guidelines for selecting, developing, comparing, and evaluating social indicators. They divide them into four categories:

1. Quality of data
2. Relation to other variables
3. Breadth of comparability
4. Usefulness

Quality of data

The characteristics of social indicators that determine the quality of the data used are as follows.

Validity. We talked about validity in Chapter 5 and must do so again here, for it is probably the baseline criterion that social indicators must meet. There are several questions that testing the validity of a social indicator must address. First of all, is an indicator conceptually or reasonably related to the reality it is proported to describe? For example, if we are interested in the amount of smoking in a population, we might use such indicators as reports of smoking behavior, cigarette sales, and morbidity and mortality rates from chronic obstructive pulmonary disease and lung cancer, which are disease conditions closely linked with smoking. Secondly, how does the indicator behave with regard to other variables that are thought to be related conceptually to the phenomenon being measured? For example, is the indicator causal, sufficient, correlated, necessary, or aggravating?[36] Aggravating indicators are those that alone are not sufficiently strong but that in company with other indicators make matters worse. Carley, referring to the concept of poverty, sees family size as a potentially aggravating indicator when coupled with low income level.[36] Alone, family size has no necessary conceptual relationship to poverty. Does the indicator predict the occurrence of an event? For example, for most of us becoming unemployed is predictive of a change in socioeconomic status. Are the sources of the data representative of the total community or population being studied? This question addresses sampling methods whether we are gathering original data or seeking to use data that have been generated by others. All of these questions need to be addressed to direct indicators, such as age, income, and housing information. Based on a number of social indicators relevant to the elderly, the instruments that were used in the two cases described in Chapters 7 and 8 were subjected to at least two kinds of validity considerations. The first, construct validity, was increased by the fact that the members of the collaborative intersystem who developed the instruments were all experienced in working with people like those to whom the questionnaires would be given or with whom the interviews would be conducted. Secondly, the actual instruments were carefully pretested with members of the elderly community with whom they would be used. Extensive changes in both format and content of the questions were made on the basis of these pretests. Validity is equally important and much more difficult to test when indirect, proxy, or surrogate indicators need be used to measure phenomena. Again, most indicators that are used to measure health are indirect ones, since the concept of health is not well defined and so direct measures are also difficult to define. Many human service workers have serious questions about the validity of the kinds of health indicators currently used, many of which focus on disease and death distributions and the use of various health services. Again, we plead for careful consideration of conceptual validity in the selection of both direct and indirect social indicators.

Reliability. Concern with reliability focuses on reducing the amount of error variance in repeated uses of the indicator with the same or similar samples. The objective of using a social indicator for comparing the occurrences of a phenomenon in a community over time is to measure changes in the phenomenon. If the instrument or indicator is reliable, one can be sure that the changes seen are indeed changes in the community and not caused by the unreliability of the instrument. Reliability is generally tested through test-retest procedures in which several uses of the indicator or measurement are made in a short period of time on comparable samples. Let us take as an example air-quality ratings. The Environmental Protection Agency has established a pollution standards index against which to compare air pollution in various cities in the United States. Reliability for these kinds of instruments is established by taking many samples of air in a given area and time and then statistically determining the variance of these tests. If the variance is too great, the instrument is refined and the test-retest procedure is repeated. In this way one can be sure, given a known variance, that the changes that show up on repeated use of indicators are caused by actual changes and not by the unreliability of the instrument itself.

Stability. Stability is similar to reliability in that it addresses an indicator's variability over time. The major differences between the two are that reliability is concerned with the consistency of the indicator, whereas stability focuses on an indicator's degree of immunity to influences such as seasons or economic changes that are conceptually irrelevant to the concept under study and the indicators used to measure it.

Responsiveness. To be useful for policy making, a social indicator must reflect changes in the phenomenon it addresses in a timely manner. For example, death rates in more developed countries or for some age groups, especially for children between 6 and 14, are less responsive indicators to sudden changes than are industrial and school absenteeism. Thus social indicators not only need to be soundly conceptually based, they also need solid grounding in the context of the total system in which they will be used. For this reason, among others, many social indicators that are appropriate for one society or cultural group are inappropriate for others. In collaboration with members of the target communities in which the indicators will be used, one can learn a great deal about the appropriateness of social indicators and so be better able to use or develop indicators that are appropriate for a given community at a particular time.

Availability of data. As we have noted before, when data are needed for almost any purpose, there is often too large or too small a supply. The wheel, or in this case the data base, should never be reinvented if it is not necessary. This means that once the collaborative planning group has a conceptualization of what the needs are and therefore what kinds of indicators are appropriate to evaluate them as a basis for decision making, they can begin to explore the available data that may address their particular interest. As we point out in the cases in Chapters 7 and 8, there were no data available on the issues the evaluations addressed and so the evaluators had little choice but to create a data base for our own decision making as well as that of everyone else. When we collect our own data, we are stuck with our own biases. These should be made clear in the report of the evaluation in terms of the limitations they place on the generalizability of the data. When we use someone else's data, we are stuck with those biases. One should know as much as possible about how these biases influence the applicability of the data to the needs one seeks to address. Given time and other resource constraints, it's terribly tempting to substitute other data that is readily available for data that one really wants but does not have access to. Unless the indicator data to be substituted clearly fit one's conceptualization of the need or problem at hand, she or he would be well advised to seek other data sources that are congruent or to develop one's own.

Scalability. Again, a major objective of social indicators is to measure relative changes in the phenomena to which they are conceptually related over time. To do this most clearly the data generated by them must not only be quantifiable but also must be scalable. This means that the data generated by the use of the indicator should be interval or ratio data. Babbie[37] clarifies the meanings of these levels of measurement. Ratio data are those whose intervals, or the distance between each unit of measurement, is the same; a measurement of zero is also possible. Thus age, length of residence in a community, level of education, and number of visits to a community facility are all ratio indicators. Interval measurements are the same as are ratio measurements except that they do not have the possibility of a measurement of zero. Fahrenheit and Celsius temperature scales are both examples of interval measurements; neither is based on absolute zero, so even though 30° Celsius is warmer than is 10° Celsius, it is not three times as warm. The data generated from Likert scales (agree to disagree) or from semantic differential scales (seven-point continuums) are ordinal measurements. The intervals on these continuums are not really equal, although we often treat them that way, nor do they have a true zero. These ordinal data are not truly scalable, as are interval and ratio data. To ensure scalability for the purposes of comparisons, the more interval and ratio measurements or indicators that can be used, the better.

Relation to other variables

Relation to other variables is the second category of the characteristics of social indicators.

Disaggregation. "All else being equal, an indicator that can be broken down by many variables tells us more about society, has a better chance of suggesting cause-and-effect relations, and is generally more valuable."[38] The Organization for Economic Cooperation and Development[39] suggests three methods that can be used to disaggregate data. We will use them to illustrate the disaggregation of infant mortal-

ity. The first is by ascribed characteristics; thus, for infant mortality one would want
to disaggregate the data by such characteristics as sex, race, and exact age of the
infants when they died. In assessing well-being characteristics, the second method,
one would want to know about mother's literacy, family income, family status or
class, and prenatal history. The third method for disaggregating indicators is in terms
of contextual variables. The kinds of contextual variables that are helpful to know in
looking at infant mortality include cause of death, location, and other infant deaths in
the locale from the same cause and at the same time. Looking at the social indicator
infant mortality from the perspectives of these component kinds of data illustrates the
value of being able to disaggregate indicator data to give a better picture of what is
really happening. We hasten to note that, again, conceptualization of the indicator
and as many of the factors that contribute to the indicator as possible is essential
before one can design the data systems that will enable one to describe the indicator
in terms of the kinds of characteristics—ascribed, well-being, and contextual—that
we have just used to illustrate the disaggregation of the social indicator infant mortality. In short, if one does not specifically seek to gather the relevant data, she or he
will not have them and so will be forced to rely on what data are available until the
needed data can be generated. This process often takes a great deal of time and other
resources.

Representativeness. Representativeness is basically a sampling process to select
a small number of social indicators that cover the essential conceptual variables with
regard to a phenomenon. Because any sampling of representative indicators, rather
than dealing with all possible indicators, results in a loss of some information; careful
conceptualization is essential to be sure that the indicators chosen to represent the
phenomenon indeed are representative. The use of representative indicators is congruent with a systems theory approach to work with communities and social indicators, since interdependence is a major concept in systems theory. However, there
are degrees of interdependence that must be carefully evaluated conceptually and
empirically so that one is sure that she or he chooses indicators that are representative of others with which they are closely interdependent and so can be assumed to
vary consistently.

Overlap with other variables. The interdependence of social indicators may be so
close as to become partially or totally overlapping. Care must be taken not to count
phenomena that are measured by more than one indicator more than once. For
example, there is some overlap between the reporting of morbidity and mortality for
serious diseases.

Breadth of comparability

Breadth of comparability is the third category of characteristics of indicators.

Intertemporal comparability. A social indicator should measure real changes over
time in the concept or phenomenon it is thought to represent. Rossi and Gilmartin[40]

give three examples of intertemporal comparability. One is that the sensitivity of the measurement may change. For example, the incidence rate of veneral diseases may seem to be increased when there is an active campaign waged to educate high-risk groups and to encourage them to seek diagnosis and treatment. The actual rate of a disease in the population may not have increased; instead what has increased is the number of people with these diseases who are seeking treatment. Changes in the population being studied may also influence the intertemporal comparability of social indicators. The increasing proportion of immigrants to the United States from Asian, African, and South American countries and the decreasing proportion of those from Europe is altering the composition of the United States population. The changes will not necessarily occur because the phenomena that the indicators measure are necessarily changing but rather because the population composition has changed and so revised indicators need to be developed. Another example is typified by changing attitudes; alcohol abuse is increasingly being thought of as a social and even a medical problem rather than as a criminal one.

Intergroup comparability. Since a major use of social indicators is to provide bases for comparisons over time and among groups, intergroup comparability should be sought. Extreme caution must be used in making comparisons among groups, among communities, or, even more complicatedly, among countries. People, cultures, environments, values, and other crucial factors that can influence indicators may vary greatly among these units of measurement. Considerable knowledge of social, cultural, and contextual characteristics of communities or other units of measurement is essential to be able to conceptualize indicators that can be used validly among them. De Neufville[41] and Murnaghan[18] illustrate many of the kinds of intergroup comparability problems in their respective discussions of developing social indicators of basic needs as guides to the United States Department of State's human rights policy and creating health indicators and information systems to facilitate efforts toward the goal of "health for all by the year 2000."[42] On a much smaller scale, we found intergroup comparability problems in our study of the elderly in four California counties as reported in Chapter 7.

Breadth of application. Indicators that can be used in a number of situations and thus permit comparisons are also desirable. Educational level is such an indicator as long as there is an understanding of what the equivalent levels of education are. Access to complete bathrooms is another, so long as the operational definition of what constitutes a complete bathroom is clear.

Usefulness

Usefulness is the fourth category of social indicator characteristics. As we discussed in Chapter 5, much of the kinds of work consultants do in collaboration with community members is in the form of some component of the evaluation process. A major reason for doing evaluations is to aid the decisions of policy makers. Since social indicators play a part in those evaluation activities, their usefulness is an important consideration.

Understandability. Social indicators are only as useful as they are understandable. Most policy makers, as well as the general public, are unfamiliar with complicated statistical techniques and terminology. Since the consultant's purpose in working with people is to help them to understand and not to bewilder them, one should find ways to translate the statistical significances, correlations, and other processes into terms the public can understand. This should not be construed to mean that consultants are not also obligated to educate people, we certainly are. However, in the process of educating them to new concepts, we must be sure that we understand both process and outcomes.

Normative interest. Social indicators that measure components of the quality of life are among those that are given normative values. Normative value means that a change in one direction is seen as "good" or desirable; a change in another direction is seen as "bad" or undesirable. For example, all other things being equal, an increased unemployment rate is seen as bad; a decrease as good. An increase in housing starts is generally seen as good; a decrease as bad. Thus, the operational definition of the desired direction of the change in an indicator is predicated on its conceptualization.

Policy relevance. Policy relevance might more accurately be called *policy potential* or *feasibility*, since it has to do with having social indicators that address issues or phenomena about which policy actions can be realistically undertaken. Despite the increasing problems with alcohol abuse, especially in young people, there is little possibility that prohibition policies will be reintroduced. In other instances, policy alternatives that are suggested by social indicators are either too time consuming or too expensive to implement. With the shortage of resources for any kind of community evaluation, one would be well advised to concentrate on developing and using indicators that address needs where there is a reasonable feasibility that the data will influence policies. There is a major exception to all of this; when one seek to raise the levels of consciousness of the public and the policy makers about a phenomenon with the idea of creating sufficient pressures to render the infeasibility of action less problematic than the consequences of inaction.

Timeliness. Timing is always important. Old data may be worse than no data at all. Policy makers need current information on which to base their decisions. Thus the quality, the quantity, and the expense of gathering relevant data need to be considered in light of the criterion of recency. This is especially true when one is seeking to evaluate concurrent changes in some social indicator.

As one works with communities and begins to develop her or his own indicators to describe and eventually, if one is careful, to be able to predict changes in social phenomena, one needs to consider all of these characteristics that sound social indicators should have. Again we stress as we have throughout this discussion that the way one conceptualizes and operationally defines both the needs that one seeks to evaluate and the social indicators that one chooses to use will greatly influence the entire process. Fig. 5 illustrates the relationship of conceptual levels, functions, and data types. Each of the three variables is numbered from 1 to 3 in ascending order of complexity. Thus most consultants start on a more or less atheoretical basis and must rely on the kinds of data that are already available in communities for initial assessments. The best one can hope to do under these circumstances is to describe what is happening within the limits of both the available data and the relative lack of theoretical basis.

Once we have lived through this stage and have learned a great deal in so doing, we as consultants are generally better able to conceptualize the needs of the community from a theoretical point of view as well as on the basis of the evaluations already completed. At that point we have a much better idea of the

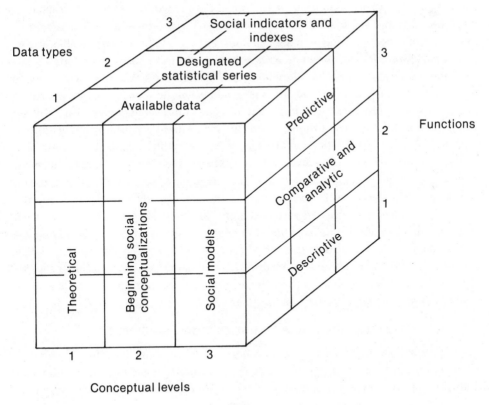

FIG. 5
Relationship of conceptual levels, functions, and data types.

kinds of data needed and can begin to design specific statistical series that will enable us to compare and analyze situations and changes in target communities or over time. This second level in the relationships of these three variables is where many community planning departments are at the present time. Almost all of the data in such publications as *Social Indicators III*[34] are these kinds of designed statistical series.

The stage in the relationship of these three variables toward which consultants need to strive is illustrated by the third variable in the figure. Sophisticated conceptualizations foster the development of social models that are both theoretically and empirically sound. The data needed for and used in these social models is at the level of social indicator and even social indices, of which we shall soon speak. These advanced levels of conceptualization and data enable policy makers to predict changes and therefore to develop much more effective policies.

Again, for those who believe that planned social change is not only possible but desirable, this final stage is a very positive one indeed. It is one that many planners, administrators, and other policy makers throughout the world are striving to achieve. For those to whom any kind of planned change or social intervention is a curse, this third level of conceptual and actual social intervention is to be avoided at all costs. As consultants work in collaboration with counterparts from many segments of target communities, we must be alert to the different values that they will bring to the collaborative intersystem and that these values will influence even as apparently straightforward a process as deciding what measures of social phenomena are needed and how to go about getting them. All of this makes life very interesting at times.

You will have noted by now that we have said very little about statistical procedures and social indicators. Statistical procedures such as multivariate analysis, analysis of variance, correlational analysis, chi-square, and multiple regression are all useful in the social indicator field, as they are in other areas, to clarify the extent of relationships between variables and indicators. However, they are useful only after these relationships have been conceptually specified. Statistical manipulations of data are not substitutes for sound conceptualization. We suggest that when you are conceptually ready to begin work with real data that you then find a statistician consultant who can assist you in the appropriate use of these methods as they relate to your conceptualizations and to your setting.

SYSTEMS APPROACH TO USE OF SOCIAL INDICATORS

Figure 6 illustrates a systems approach to the use of social indicators in community planning and evaluating processes. The input into the community planning and evaluating subsystem is a number of different kinds of indicators, other input of various kinds, and feedback from the process, its outcomes, and its consequences. We give some objective and subjective, or quantitative and qualitative, indicators under each of the indicator headings by way of example.

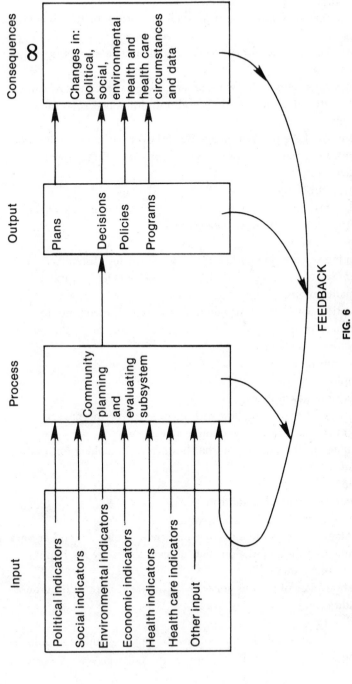

FIG. 6

Systems model of community planning and evaluating processes using indicators.

Political indicators
1. Voting patterns especially in local elections
2. Participation in political groups such as parties or the League of Women Voters
3. Proportion of special interest and other aggregate members in appointed and elected positions
4. People's satisfaction with government, especially local government
5. People's attitudes towards their ability to influence government

Social indicators
1. Percentage of the population age 25 and over without a high school diploma
2. Percentage of the population who do not speak English well or at all
3. Homicide rate
4. Feelings of belonging
5. Level of fear reported by the people in various neighborhoods
6. Perceptions of community cohesiveness

Environmental indicators
1. Percentage of the population with a work-related disability
2. Percentage of dwellings with 1.01 or more persons per room
3. Air-quality ratings
4. Satisfaction with the environmental quality of the community
5. Percentage of the population who would recommend the community as a good environment in which to live

Economic indicators
1. Unemployment rate
2. Number of bankruptcies
3. Percentage of the population with income below the poverty level
4. Level of satisfaction with economic status
5. Percentage of the population that has given up looking for a job

Health indicators
1. Suicide rate
2. Elementary school absenteeism
3. Death rate for cirrhosis of the liver
4. Percentage of the population that rate their health as good or very good
5. Percentage of the population that indicate that they are happy

Health care indicators
1. Utilization rates of various services by different population groups
2. Morbidity rate
3. Mortality rate
4. Number, location, and types of institutional, group, and solo health care providers

5. People's perceptions of the availability of health care
6. People's perceptions of the acceptability of health care
7. People's perceptions of the affordability of health care

These lists are in no way exhaustive, but they do illustrate some of the variety of quantitative and qualitative indicators that can be used as input into the community's planning and evaluating subsystem. The collaborative planning or evaluating group must decide what indicators are conceptually relevant for their use and then operationally define each one before beginning to gather and use data.

The community planning and evaluating subsystem uses the indicator data that it has defined as relevant and needed as a basis for its processes. Obviously many of the kinds of output that the community planning and evaluating subsystem will produce are based on political and other pragmatic considerations as well as on the basis of the indicator data. As noted earlier, the data may clearly pinpoint needed action, but political and other constraints may preclude meaningful changes. Although this is frustrating, particularly for those who have a vested interest in the phenomena the data address, it is a reality of community life and must be expected. This expectation enables one to make contingency plans that sometimes can alter these realities at least to some degree.

Output that the community planning and evaluation subsystem produces includes plans for subsequent actions, decisions between alternative courses of action, policies that serve as guides to actions, and actions themselves such as programs or other kinds of services. The consequences of this output are reflected in changes in the same indicator data that were types of input at the beginning of the cycle. These consequences continue on into infinity. They are a major source of feedback to the community planning and evaluating subsystem, and so the system continues.

This model illustrates the importance of indicator data to the functioning of the community planning and evaluating subsystem. It also illustrates why indicator data must be comparably collected over periods of time to enable measurements of changes or consequences that are influenced by the output of the subsystem's processes. In addition, it clearly shows the interdependence of all parts of the system.

Before leaving the model and its variety of indicator data, we need to comment about the uses of quantitative (or objective) and qualitative (or subjective) indicators. In each of the lists of indicators, we have given examples of both those that can be objectively observed and counted and those that must be sought in different ways. Since most of the data with which consultants work are quantitative, or objective, they are more familiar with them. Qualitative, or subjective, data are equally important, particularly when they are dealing with evaluations of quality of life. As Carley[43] points out, "For most researchers, however, quality-of-life research means attention to subjective social indicators."

Qualitative indicators, as our examples illustrate, deal with people's perceptions, attitudes, beliefs, and descriptions of their experiences. Combined or aggregated, these subjective data provide an essential dimension about services, environment, living conditions, and other phenomena for use in planning and evaluating. *Subjective data* is a term preferred by some; however, since they are often assigned numerical values and quantified, the term can lead to another semantic swamp. Subjective data must be designed and generated with the same attention to their quality as one gives to the gathering of objective data. All of the research and evaluation skills discussed in Chapter 5 are very much needed in working with subjective social indicators. The products are worth the effort.

SOCIAL INDICES

Dever defines a health status index as, "A composite measure which summarizes data from two or more components (variables) and which, like an indicator, also purports to reflect the health status of an individual or defined group."[44] This same definition can be readily applied to any index. He suggests that the following four questions should be answered in the development of an index:[45]

1. What is the purpose of the index? This is by now the very familiar question about the conceptual basis for the development and use of the index. What is the index supposed to measure and how will it do so?
2. What are the exact components of the index? Since an index is a composite of several variables, these variables must be clearly defined and must fit into the conceptualization of the index. Variables for inclusion must also be carefully and exactly operationally defined.
3. What is the form of interpretation? This is the analysis and use question regarding the index. What assumptions of statistical tests do the data for the index meet and therefore which statistical computations are appropriate?
4. What are the limitations of the index? No index is perfect and so one must be clear in recognizing and considering the index's limitations. Many feel that all indices are severely limited as a result of both conceptual and methodological inadequacies.[46,47]

Sackett and others[48] present seven prerequisites for health indices; these, too, are equally applicable to all indices:

1. *Comprehensiveness.* Indices must embrace a broad spectrum of relevant variables that are thought by experts to be both representative and comparable.
2. *Positive orientation.* Indices should need to focus on good or even excellent functions as well as on negative ones. This is a particularly important prerequisite for health indices, since most so-called health indicator data focus on disease, disablity, and death rather than on health.
3. *General applicability.* Variables used in the index should be applicable to many groups to enable comparisons to be made within and among groups.

4. *Sensitivity.* The variables that make up the index must be sensitive or responsive enough to enable the index to reflect changes in a timely manner.
5. *Simplicity, acceptability, and cost.* This prerequisite addresses the ever-
present constraint of resources, as well as the needs for the index to be
understandable and relatively easily constructed, preferably from existing
data, if the conceptual basis for their use is sound.
6. *Precision.* This again concerns validity and reliability. Index construction
must be even more concerned with these criteria than is indicator construction, since aggregation of a number of indicators into an index can also result
in aggregation of their individual shortcomings. As a result, the index could
become very misleading.
7. *Amenability to index construction.* The indicators included would have to be
in a form that enables rapid combination. For this reason subjective data
or objective data requiring substantial content analysis are less applicable to
index construction than are objective data based on counts of the incidence or
the prevalence of phenomena.

Physical Quality of Life Index

The Physical Quality of Life Index is an example of a social index.

The Physical Quality of Life Index was developed by Morris[28] under the aegis of
the Overseas Development Council as part of "a growing number of efforts to devise
indicators that measure progress in physical well-being more effectively than is readily possible with gross national product and other monetary indicators."[49] This reflects the past, as Carley's comment[50] about the social indicator movement in the
mid-1960s shows: "Initially this was a reaction against what was perceived as an
overemphasis on measures of economic performance as indicators of social well-
being." Recall what we said about change in Chapter 2.

The Physical Quality of Life Index is a composite of three equally weighted
indicators: infant mortality, life expectancy at age 1, and literacy rate.[28] All three have
considerable credibility as individual indicators and so have conceptual validity and
reliability. Data on all three indicators are available for all countries.

1. *Infant mortality* is on a scale of 0 to 100. The range of infant mortality is from
7 infant deaths per 1000 live births, which is one less than Sweden's rate (the
world's lowest), to 229, which is the record for any country since the United
Nations began collecting infant mortality data in the 1950s. On the scale, 7 is
assigned the value of 0, and 229, the value of 100. Thus a change in infant
mortality of 2.22 deaths per 1000 live births registers a one-point change on
the scale.
2. *Life expectancy at age 1* is based on the United Nations' data and ranges from
the lowest of 38 years to the highest of 77 years. A change of 0.39 years of life
expectancy is equal to a 1-point change on the scale of 0 to 100.

3. *Literacy rate* describes the percentage of the population 15 years of age and older that is literate. Since this indicator is a percentage, it can be transcribed directly on a scale of 0 to 100.

Some of the comments on the rationale for the Physical Quality of Life Index that Morris gives include the following:[28]

1. Worst performance (0) on the scale is clearly defined. There is a capacity to measure deterioration in even the worst rates by using negative scores as needed.
2. Best performance is also clearly defined and there is a capacity to measure improvement in even the best rates.
3. All three indicators in the Physical Quality of Life Index are equally weighted, making the index an average of the total scores of the three indicators.
4. Cross-country comparisons can be made since the indicators in the index are common to all. All countries' performances are judged on the same indicators and on an identical scale.
5. The composite scoring of the three indicators encourages the consideration of their interrelationships with the quality of life within and among countries.

Although the Physical Quality of Life Index is not without its critics, it is an elegantly simple and conceptually valid approach to looking at factors other than economic ones in developing indices for measuring and comparing the quality of life among countries.[51,52] Similar kinds of indices are badly needed to aid those who work collaboratively with community groups to evaluate the community's quality of life and to make decisions about ways to change it for the better.

SUMMARY

In this chapter we have presented a brief overview of the history and development of social indicators and the social indicator movement. We stressed throughout the need for sound conceptualization of social indicators. Social indicators were defined as statistical measurements of social conditions and their changes over time. Following the discussion of some of the kinds and uses of social indicators, we presented a number of characteristics that social indicators should have. Paramount among them are validity and reliability. Fig. 6 (p. 133) shows the relationship of conceptual levels, functions, and data types with the level toward which many people are striving, defined as social models that are the basis for the development and use of social indicators and indices for predictive purposes. Our systems model for community planning and evaluating processes show the use of a variety of indicators as input to the planning and evaluation processes as well as consequences of their outcomes. The chapter closes with a discussion of social indices and their prerequisites. The Physical Quality of Life Index is presented as a model and we urge the development of similar indices for use in community planning and evaluation.

REFERENCES

1. Barnhart, C.L., and others, editors: The American college dictionary, New York, 1970, Random House, Inc., p. 1181.
2. Brun, B.: The timetables of history: a horizontal linkage of people and events, updated ed., New York, 1979, Simon & Schuster, Inc.
3. Nectoux, F., Lintott, J., and Carr-Hill, R.: Social indicators: for individual well-being or social control? International Journal of Health Services 10(1):89-113, 1980.
4. Carley, M.: Social measurement and social indicators: issues of policy and theory, London, 1981, George Allen & Unwin, Ltd., p. 14.
5. Lazarsfeld, P.F.: Quantification in sociology. In Woolf, H., editor: Quantification, Indianapolis, 1961, The Bobbs-Merrill Co., Inc.
6. Pigou, A.C.: The economics of welfare, ed. 2, London, 1924, Macmillan, Inc.
7. Rossi, R.J., and Gilmartin, K.J.: The handbook of social indicators: sources, characteristics, and analyses, New York, 1980, Garland STPM Press.
8. Rossi and Gilmartin, p. 2.
9. Brauer, R.A., editor: Social indicators, Cambridge, Mass., 1966, The MIT Press.
10. Sheldon, E.B., and Moore, W.E., editors: Indicators of social change: concepts and measurements, New York, 1968, Russell Sage Foundation.
11. Campbell, A., and Converse, P.E., editors: The human meaning of social change, New York, 1972, Russell Sage Foundation.
12. Land, K.C., and Silverman, S., editors: Social indicator models, New York, 1975, Russell Sage Foundation.
13. Duncan, O.D.: Toward social reporting: next steps. In Social science frontiers, no. 2, New York, 1969, Russell Sage Foundation.
14. Rossi and Gilmartin, p. 9-10.
15. Organization for Economic Cooperation and Development, Directorate for Manpower and Social Affairs: List of social concerns common to most OECD countries: the OECD social indicator development program, Washington, D.C., 1973, OECD Publications Center.
16. Organization for Economic Cooperation and Development: Measuring social well-being: a progress report on the development of social indicators, Washington, D.C., 1976, OECD Publications Center.
17. United Nations Statistical Office: A system of demographic, manpower, and social statistics series, classification, and social indicators, New York, 1971, United Nations.
18. Murnaghan, J.H.: Health indicators and information systems for the year 2000. In Breslow, L., editor: Annual review of public health, vol. 2, Palo Alto, Calif. 1981, Annual Reviews, Inc., pp. 299-361.
19. Carley, pp. 12-14.
20. Census of Population and Housing: Summary characteristics for government units and SMSAs, Washington, D.C., 1982, U.S. Department of Commerce, Bureau of Census.
21. De Nuefville, J.: Social indicators and public policy: interactive processes of design and application, New York, 1975, Elsevier Scientific Publishing Co., p. 121.
22. Carlisle, E.: The conceptual structure of social indicators. In Schonfield, A., and Shaw, S., editors: Social indicators and social policy, London, 1972, Heinemann Educational Books, pp. 25-27.
23. Rossi and Gilmartin, p. 56.
24. Land, K.: Theories, models, and indicators of social change, International Social Science Journal 27:14, 1975.

25. Fanchette, S.: Social indicators: problems of methodology and selection. In Social indicators: problems of methodology and selection, Paris, 1974, United Nations Education, Social, and Cultural Organization, p. 8.
26. Carley, p. 28.
27. Murnaghan, p. 303.
28. Morris, M.D.: Measuring the condition of the world's poor: the physical quality of life index, New York, 1979, Pergamon Press.
29. Streeten, P., and others: First things first: meeting basic human needs in developing countries, New York, 1981, Oxford University Press.
30. Archer, S.E., and Fleshman, R.P.: Selected concepts for client-centered community health nursing. In Community health nursing: patterns and practice, ed. 3, N. Scituate, Mass., Duxbury Press. (In press.)
31. Land, p. 14.
32. Snider, E.L.: Social indicators, health policy, and the elderly, Social Indicators Research 11:405-419, 1982.
33. Patton, M.O.: Qualitative evaluation methods, Beverly Hills, Calif., 1980, Sage Publications, Inc.
34. Social Indicators III: Selected data on social conditions and trends in the United States, Washington, D.C., 1980, U.S. Department of Commerce, Bureau of the Census, Center for Demographic Studies.
35. Rossi and Gilmartin, pp. 33-47.
36. Carley, p. 32.
37. Babbie, E.R.: Survey research methods, Belmont, Calif., 1973, Wadsworth Publishing Co., Inc., pp. 138-140.
38. Rossi and Gilmartin, p. 38.
39. Organization for Economic Cooperation and Development, pp. 30-40.
40. Rossi and Gilmartin, p. 40.
41. de Neufville, J.I.: Social indicators of basic needs: quantitative data for human rights policy, Social Indicators Research 11:383-403, 1982.
42. World Health Organization/United Nations International Children's Emergency Fund: Primary health care, report of the International Conference on Primary Health Care, Alma Ata, USSR, Geneva, September 1978, World Health Organization.
43. Carley, p. 34.
44. Dever, G.E.A.: Community health analysis: a holistic approach, Germantown, Md., 1980, Aspen Systems Corp., p. 177.
45. Dever, p. 193.
46. Health Status Indexes Conference, Health Services Research, vol. 11, Winter 1976, p. 340.
47. Murnaghan, p. 304.
48. Sackett, D.L., and others: The development and application of indices of health: general methods and a summary of results, American Journal of Public Health 67:423-424, May 1977.
49. Grant, J.P.: Forward. In Morris, p. xi.
50. Carley, p. 1.
51. Murnaghan, p. 304.
52. Jaeger-Burns, J.: The relationship of nursing to primary health internationally, Int. Nurs. Rev. 28:167-175, 1981.

7

SENIOR LIFE-STYLE SURVEY

In this chapter and in Chapter 8 we discuss the background, planning, implementation, and outcomes of two cross-sectional evaluations that we conducted in northern California. The target aggregate in both evaluations was the elderly population living within a defined community.

Much of our focus is on the collaborative processes involved in the conduct of these two evaluations and on the problems we encountered in carrying them out. Most reports of studies of this kind give little attention to how they were actually done. Few discuss the problems and frustrating facets of this kind of work. We need to know about these before we begin so that we can anticipate at least some of the pitfalls, even if we cannot avoid them. Some of the problems we faced include: defining the target aggregate to be studied, determining what to study and what not to study, gaining access to the target aggregate and then to the actual subjects, dealing with gatekeepers, and the fact that investigators often have to pay dues or earn the right to have access to the target aggregate. Although we do not have solutions for all of these problems, we offer the strategies we used to cope with them as examples of what others can do as well. We write here with the clarity of "20-20 hindsight."

Nursing Dynamics Corporation (NDC) did the first evaluation described in this Chapter from 1975 to 1976. The purpose of this needs assessment was to gather baseline data on the needs and wants of the socially active elderly aggregate in four suburban and rural California counties. We were also interested in selected dimensions of their health status and life styles. At the time we conducted the study there were no baseline data available from the elderly *themselves* for use by planners and service providers to develop appropriate resources for the elderly. Our client organi-

---

Throughout this chapter *we* refers to Sarah Archer and Ruth Fleshman, the principal investigators, and Lannie Adelman and Carol Carver, research assistants. In this chapter and in Chapter 8, identifying information such as names of places and agencies have been changed to maintain confidentiality.

zation with which we collaborated for this needs assessment was the Area Agency on Aging (AAA) that at that time served the four communities we studied. The AAA is the community subsystem that planned and coordinated services for the elderly.

NEEDS AND LIFE-STYLE ASSESSMENT OF COMMUNITY ELDERLY, 1975-1976
Background

At the time we undertook this assessment, NDC[1] had been working with the elderly aggregate in a suburban northern California community for 2 years. Our efforts at that time were entirely focused on health promotion and primary prevention to help the well elderly to maintain their optimal level of functioning.[2]

Seeking information about our elderly clients' needs from a variety of sources such as the comprehensive health planning agency, the AAA, the city and community planning departments, and other community agencies that also worked with the elderly aggregate turned up very little data that we could use to plan and develop the kinds of services that would meet the needs of the elderly. Therefore we had little option but to undertake to gather this kind of baseline data ourselves. We were encouraged to do so by many of our colleague agencies in the community, who also needed the data that would be generated by such an assessment and so were very eager to collaborate in this needs assessment.

Funding for such an assessment is always difficult to obtain. None of our collaborating agencies could help with money or computer capabilities, so we turned to other sources. Sarah Archer was able to obtain funding through the School of Nursing at the University of California at San Francisco Biomedical Research Support Grant, to pay the meager salaries of two of her graduate students in community health nursing and gerontology to work as research assistants on the project. Because graduate students were involved in the data processing, the University also provided computer time. With these slim resources in hand, we were able to begin. Sarah Archer donated her time as part of her community service commitment from the University, and Ruth Fleshman donated her time as part of her responsibilities as president of NDC. We began the study early in 1975 and completed the report late in 1976. During the study we visited almost 100 senior sites and activities, had uncounted meetings with colleagues and agency staff, and collected 679 usable responses from well elderly participants. It all sounds easy and clean from the perspective of several years away. However, the actual process was neither clean nor easy.

Assessment design

We used a descriptive cross-sectional design in that we looked at our respondents in one time period rather than longitudinally (see Chapter 5). After considerable investigation, we learned that the only complete listing of people 65 and over that existed at the time we were considering sampling methodology was the Social Security list. On inquiry at the Social Security office, we learned that *no one* outside of the Social Security office itself was given access to the list of seniors' names and addresses. Even though we were working with a community agency, the AAA, on county business, we could not use the list. As evaluators, we were concerned and even dismayed since this decision meant that we had no hope of doing a random sample of the elderly community aggregate. However, as providers of services to elderly clients, we were relieved to know that this kind of protection for their privacy existed, even from us "insiders." Since random sampling was not possible and because there was no other systematic way to reach the elderly target aggregate, we had no choice but to use a convenience sample. This sample consisted of those well elderly people who attended senior center or senior club activities or who took their noon meal at one of the title VII (Older Americans' Act) dining sites and who volunteered to participate. We could find no other way to gain access to the numbers of seniors we wanted to invite to participate in the assessment. A convenience sample, because it is in no way a random selection of participants, limits the generalizability of the findings. We sought to reduce this limitation by seeking increases in the number of respondents (n = 679).

Instrument construction. We chose a self-administered anonymous questionnaire that we developed for this assessment (see pp. 153-158 and Chapter 5). We believed that this instrument was preferable to individual interviews for several reasons.

1. The literacy rate among our target aggregate of active elderly was known to be quite high. Thus we were confident that our respondents would be able to read and understand the questionnaire and to write down their own answers for us. Actually, only one individual had to have the assessment done as an interview because he could not read English.

2. Because we had been doing health counseling and health promotion activities with well elderly people for several years, we had had opportunities to gather in-depth information on life-style, health care needs, and wants from our individual clients. Thus we had a great deal of field data from our individual clients that we could use to develop items for the questionnaire. We were confident that questions so developed and administered would elicit the breadth of information we sought from the assessment. We also sought input from members of collaborating agencies.

3. Questionnaires are much less expensive to administer than are one-to-one interviews. Given our limited personnel, money, and time available for the assessment, the questionnaire format enabled us to get the most information for our limited resources.

4. Because of the reality that we would use a convenience sample, the questionnaire format not only enabled us to reach more people, it allowed them to protect their privacy and anonymity. Often extremely personal or sensitive information can be elicited with less trauma for the subject through an impersonal medium such as a self-administered questionnaire than can be obtained through an interview.

Questionnaires and other written materials given to elderly respondents must be written in large type and be well spaced so that they can be read easily by persons whose visual acuity is impaired. Otherwise, especially on a long instrument such as ours, respondents may tire and give up before finishing all the questions. We learned this on the pretest and so could develop the final instrument appropriately.

We developed the survey instrument in collaboration with other experts in the field of aging as well as with considerable review of the literature to ensure construct and face validity. Pretesting also helped us to refine the language in the questions, to weed out health jargon and "nursespeak," and to be sure respondents could understand what we were asking them. We put the instrument through three successive pretests with members of the well elderly aggregate. Each time we revised the questions according to their suggestions. In this way we arrived at an instrument that we were fairly confident potential respondents would be able to understand and to answer. This kind of assurance of validity is essential if gathered data are to be useful.

In spite of these efforts, we still found that some of the questions were confusing to respondents. We judged this from the frequency of their requests for interpretation of the questions as well as from the number of times that the problem questions were skipped completely, were partially answered, or were answered in ways that led us to believe that our meaning had been unclear. Questions 2 and 52 (see Instrument, p. 153 and p. 158) were particularly problematic. Those of us who grew up with Likert-type scales are accustomed to them. People who are not familiar with these kinds of scales often have difficulties with them. We avoided ranking questions because of our experience that people have considerable trouble ordering alternatives. These kinds of problems must be considered as consultants select the question formats they want to use.

Another problem question was 31, where we asked what kinds of conditions respondents either thought they had (i.e., they had self-diagnosed) or conditions that physicians had told them they had. Many respondents seemed to have difficulty differentiating these two kinds of diagnoses on the questionnaire, although in health counseling interviews elderly clients could clearly say that they thought they had a given condition such as arthritis even if they had not been formally diagnosed by a physician as having it. Finally, some respondents will select more than one answer to a question even if the directions clearly and repeatedly state that only one answer or the best answer is to be chosen.

The instrument, as a quick look on pp. 153-158 will show, was very long and involved. We succumbed to the all-too-frequent temptation to ask everything we wanted to know all at once. Had we had the resources, a far better approach would have been to spread the questions over several assessments. In this way we might have obtained better data on a limited number of questions. There is always a trade-off between what needs to be done and the amount of resources available to do it. The problem of length was complicated by the fact that virtually every collaborating agency begged to have us ask their pet question. One must carefully weigh the requests of other agencies and providers to include their questions when length is a concern. However, adding a few extra questions may pay big dividends in terms of data and in gaining goodwill and future cooperation from other providers. This is an example of another trade-off.

Once you have done the best you can to ensure that your instrument is as appropriate, valid, and reliable as possible, you are ready to start. Now the real fun of interacting with respondents and gathering data begins.

Preparing investigators. Four community health nurses conducted this assessment and authored the report, which can be found at the end of this chapter. As noted, Ruth Fleshman and Sarah Archer were both involved because of their affiliation with NDC and with the university. Through the University of California School of Nursing, Sarah Archer was able to obtain funds to pay two graduate students in community health nursing and gerontology, Carole Carver and Lannie Adelman, to also work on the study. The four evaluators worked closely together to develop the assessment and the logistics of its conduct. All four were experienced community health nurses who had worked with the elderly. All had expertise in working with groups and in providing health education programs; skills that were to prove very useful in gaining access to many groups of potential respondents.

Together the four evaluators prepared the explanatory speech each would give to introduce and discuss the purpose of the assessment and the uses to which the data would be put. Since the assessment instrument was a self-administered questionnaire, the kind of practicing and standardizing that would have been required had the instrument been an interview was less critical. What we sought instead was to ensure that each investigator introduced and explained the assessment and process in the same way. This uniform presentation helped to reduce bias or skew that could have resulted if each investigator explained the study to potential respondents in a different manner.

We all met at regular intervals after data collection was begun to share experiences, to discuss questions that respondents raised, to agree on uniform answers to the kinds of questions raised, and to try to anticipate problems. We were fortunate in this assessment to have experienced investigators. Special attention was given to assuring that the graduate students understood as much about what was going on as possible. This was seen as a vital part of their educational experience in working on the assessment.[3] All of us shared in the fun of the evaluation as well as in the problems and drudgery involved. We wanted everyone's participation in the assessment to be more than just another valuable learning experience.

Informed consent. The ethics of conducting any kind of research that involves human subjects requires that the subjects understand what they are being asked to participate in, what the purposes of the study are, what the risks and benefits to them are, and the measures the evaluators have taken to reduce the risks for respondents (see Chapter 5). Because community evaluations such as the ones we are describing here involve people, informed consent must be sought from potential respondents.

One of the evaluators took the questionnaires to the senior center, senior club, or dining site; explained the purpose of the study; described how the data would be analyzed and repeated; and asked members of the group to voluntarily participate. Each presenter stressed that participation was totally voluntary, that respondents would not be compensated in any way, that the decisions of persons to participate or not to participate would in no way influence their eligibility for any service offered by any agency, that data would be presented in such a way that no one could be identified even by him or herself, and that those who chose to participate could decide to stop filling out the questionnaire anytime they wished to or could skip any question. In this way we did as much as we could to inform them about the nature of the study and the means that we had and would take to preserve their anonymity and reduce any social risk for them. We offered to answer individual questions about the questionnaire or the study in general.

In addition, we offered to provide anyone in the groups with individual health counseling and referral services if they wished to make their needs known to us. A number did so, and we worked with them as needed. We asked that they contact us directly or hand us a note separate from the questionnaire to preserve their anonymity on the instrument. We stressed repeatedly that they should not identify themselves in any way on the questionnaire. We did not use a formal consent form that would have required a participant's signature. Instead we assumed the individual's consent to participate if she or he completed any of the items on the questionnaire. This decision was another means of ensuring anonymity.

Administration of the instrument. We chose to have one of the evaluators take the questionnaires to the site for administration, do the explanation, answer questions, distribute the questionnaires, provide or arrange for needed health counseling and referrals, and collect the questionnaires herself. This ensured uniformity of presentation as a basis for informed consent to participate and personal contact with respondents, and it increased the probability that questionnaires would be returned to us. Although more expensive in evaluator time and gasoline than mailing the questionnaires would have been, we felt that the advantages of having one of us talk directly with potential respondents, answer questions, and personally conduct the study far outweighed the disadvantages. It also greatly improved the response rate. This decision also proved to be very effective because one of us was on hand to answer questions, a fact that improved the quality of the data we got back and ensured that questionnaires were returned to us. One of us was also available to offer counseling and referral services on request. There were two exceptions to this procedure. At the senior center where NDC had been providing health counseling for some time, we had worked with and trained several senior volunteers who were as interested in and as capable as we were to administer and collect the questionnaires. One of the evaluators worked closely with these women and was available to answer their questions as the need arose. The other exception was not nearly so successful. In a few instances in the three communities to which the study was extended toward the end, members of the senior center, club, or dining site staff administered the questionnaires. Both the quality and the quantity of responses under these circumstances were less than when one of the evaluators was able to be present. This aspect is further discussed later.

Finding people to assess: access and entry

We began this assessment of the well elderly aggregate in NDC's home community. Members of the NDC had been working with members of the elderly group in health counseling for 2 years. We who were members of NDC were familiar to providers, to agencies, and to the elderly themselves either through personal contact with us or via word of mouth. In short, NDC had begun to establish credibility in our local community, with our peer providers, and with our real and potential clients. Thus the evaluator and community systems were already familiar with each other. The collaborative evaluation intersystem for this evaluation was therefore quickly and effectively established. This collaborative intersystem planned the assessment, developed the instrument, and sought feedback constantly from both community and consultant systems. This feedback enabled us to make needed changes in the assessment as we went along (see Chapter 5). In addition, this credibility made both access and entry easier in our own community than was to be the case later when the assessment was expanded to three adjacent rural counties where NDC had less of a track record.

The target aggregate for this assessment was the socially active well elderly in the county. We chose this aggregate because the people in it were those in whom we were interested and with whom we had already begun to work in health education and health counseling. To take advantage of the economies of scale, we sought out sites where groups of potential respondents for the assessment gathered. We contacted the staff of the various senior clubs, senior centers, and title VII dining sites throughout the county, explained the study to them, and asked permission to come to their site during a meeting or at meal time to talk about the assessment with the senior participants and to invite their participation. Our greatest problem in our own community was to obtain a scheduled time on the agendas of the senior groups. We had to compete with luncheons, business meetings, other speakers, field trips, bingo and card games, bowling leagues, and an endless array of other recreational and educational activities. The people we sought were really active elderly, and to find the 60 to 90 minutes needed to discuss and conduct our assessment in their busy schedules was a challenge. Through both perseverance and patience we succeeded, although more than a year of data gathering was required to do so. These kinds of negotiations for access take a great deal of time, so be sure to allow for them in your planning of the assessment program (see Fig. 2, p. 32).

Once people knew that one of the evaluators was coming to a meeting or meal anyway, they often asked that she give a short health education program. We welcomed these opportunities because they enabled us to talk with people about ways to promote and to maintain their health. Since our major objective in our work with the elderly was health promotion and maintenance, we welcomed invitations to provide these kinds of programs to any group who would listen to them. These presentations also "paid" in a way for people's participation in the assessment—trade-offs are everywhere.

One of the evaluators went through the procedure presented earlier in the discussion of administration of the instrument. The whole process of administering the questionnaire to one group of seniors often took at least half a day, including travel to and from the site. This time frame did not include the preplanning and scheduling time nor the time for follow-up on referral and other requests that our presentation generated. Obviously, coding the questionnaires and preparing the data for the computer also required substantial additional time. Community assessments are not quick to do if one is doing them in any depth.

Expansion of the assessment to three rural communities

Once we were well along with the assessment in NDC's home community, the members of the collaborative intersystem began to discuss the pros and cons of extending the assessment to the three rural communities under the AAA's jurisdiction. The AAA's rationale for the request to expand the assessment was that there were even less data available on seniors' needs and life-styles in these three rural communities than was the case in NDC's suburban home community. Members of the collaborative intersystem agreed to expand the assessment. The AAA gave us a blanket endorsement and introductions to the staff of all the senior centers, senior clubs, and title VII dining sites in the three rural communities. This gives the impression that we had clear sailing from then on; however, that was not the case.

Some very critical dimensions for conducting a community assessment were missing for the investigators in the three rural communities. The three rural communities were much less cohesive themselves and so it was difficult to draw representatives from those communities into the collaborative evaluation intersystem. We tried but were less successful than we wanted to be for several reasons. Although Ruth Fleshman and Sarah Archer had done some health education programs and consultation for the AAA in the three rural counties, NDC was unknown as an agency and so had no credibility with either local providers or potential respondents. The AAA itself was less active and therefore less influential in these communities. This was partially because these counties had fewer elderly residents and they were more scattered. Rural people, particularly rural elderly people, tend to be conservative. They are often more fiercely self-reliant—by necessity if not by choice—than are many urban or suburban elderly. At least partially for this reason, the people in the three rural counties were more reluctant or reticent to participate in the assessment than were the people in the suburban community.

People in the suburban county, who were physically closer to the University of California at San Francisco, were more familiar·with the university's public service work in its surrounding communities. Thus they were more accepting of the university's involvement in the study through the School of Nursing. The elderly people in the rural counties seemed much more suspicious of the university's involvement, a factor that influenced some potential respondent's willingness to participate. Thus, a word of caution needs to be emphasized here about selecting an agency or agencies to collaborate in a community assessment. Collaborating groups' reputations can lend prestige and credibility to the assessment; they can also adversely affect it, especially in terms of peoples' willingness to participate. Investigators must consider the trade-offs between the pros and cons of choosing to collaborate with other agencies or groups.

In retrospect, the expansion of the assessment to the three rural counties was probably unwise for the reasons already given. In addition, we found ourselves overextended. For example, the distance between NDC's headquarters or the University to assessment sites in the three rural counties was over 100 miles round trip. Even when access could be gained to senior sites in these three counties, the numbers of people at the various sites at any one time was often much smaller than was the case in the suburban community. Thus, we encountered many diseconomies of scale; the results did not justify the efforts.

As a result of the decision of the collaborative evaluation intersystem to expand the assessment to the three rural communities, the evaluators found that we were spending a great deal more time and were traveling substantial distances to obtain relatively small returns in terms of the numbers of completed questionnaires that resulted. Another less than optimum decision made by the collaborative evaluation intersystem in an attempt to reduce the diseconomies of scale for the evaluators was to have some of the staff at the various senior centers, clubs, and dining sites in the three rural communities to conduct the assessment themselves and to mail the completed questionnaires back to us. Generally, we did this with reluctance and at their insistence. It also meant we had to orient them to the specific format of the conduct of the assessment. Even though many of the staff were cooperative and conscientious, others were less so. The results obtained reflected these variations in the staff members' commitment to the project. It is unrealistic to expect, that with few exceptions people not vitally involved with a community assessment will devote the same energy and concern to its conduct as do members of the collaborative evaluation intersystem. This therefore proved to be another valuable learning experience.

Gatekeepers. By far the greatest problem of access in the three rural communities was the role of gatekeeper that many of the members of senior center, senior club, and dining site staff elected to play. They effectively kept us from reaching their groups of seniors by denying us permission to come to sites at a time when the seniors were there. We are sure that these staff members believed that they were looking after the best interests of their elderly constituents. In reality, they were making the decision for them instead of permitting the seniors to make their own decisions after we had had an opportunity to talk with them. As a result, we faced the challenge of selling the assessment to the staff of the senior sites before we could even talk with the seniors themselves. To say the least, many of the staff in the three rural communities were unenthusiastic about the project. Again perhaps because they had not been directly involved in planning it. This is interesting in light of the fact that after our presentations, when we were able to gain access to the seniors themselves, approximately 80% of those present completed at least some of the questionnaire.

To be sure, we realized that we have to cope as effectively as possible with these gatekeepers. Often the staff people at the various sites in the rural communities wanted to meet with one or more of the evaluators and to see the assessment tool before they would even consider the possibility of scheduling its presentation at their sites. Whenever possible the investigators, through the AAA or independently, attempted to arrange for representatives to meet with us at one time. In this way we sought to conserve resources. The fact remained that each of these meetings with staff took at least one of the investigators virtually a full day to conduct. This should be no surprise since the geographical area this assessment covered had grown to approximately 2000 square miles. We have not been either so ambitious or foolhardy again. In desperation and often against our better judgment, as noted, we occasionally consented to permit the staff members to conduct the assessment for us, usually with less than optimum results.

Assessing men. A final access problem in this aggregate assessment was to reach a representative proportion of elderly men. Most of the people attending senior centers, clubs, and dining sites in our target areas were women. This is reflected in the fact that 79% of our respondents were women. We knew that in 1975 and 1976 approximately 40% of the population over 65 was male. Thus, elderly men are seriously underrepresented in our assessment. Elderly men are generally married and living with their spouses. As such, they are less likely than are elderly women, who are more frequently widowed or never married, to be present at many of the kinds of sites where we sought our convenience sample. We made repeated efforts to gain entry to the all-male senior club in our home county; however, all attempts were unsuccessful. The staff and officers of the group simply had more important things to schedule than the evaluation we proposed. Actually, NDC was never able to gain access to members of this group for any purpose, nor were most other agencies. Of course, we respected their decision, even though it precluded our reaching the largest concentration of elderly men in the county.

Analysis of data

Data from the 679 respondents in this assessment were coded and prepared for computer tabulation and analysis as described in Chapter 5. We used the Statistical Package for the Social Sciences (SPSS),[4] which was available at the University of

California at San Francisco's campus. Closed-ended questions such as questions 1 through 5 (see the questionnaire on pp. 153-158) were easy to code and tabulate. Open-ended questions such as 6, 12, and 14 were another matter.

The four evaluators worked together to develop the codebook for the open-ended questions. After about 100 completed questionnaires had been accumulated, we all read through the answers for each open-ended question, made our initial categorization of the answers, discussed our categories for the answers to the open-ended questions to assess our interrater reliability, and finally agreed on the array of responses that we would use to code each open-ended question.

Once the codebook was prepared, we were able to code the questionnaires after each administration. As questions arose or new categories of answers to open-ended questions emerged, we discussed them and came to an agreement on how they should be coded. The graduate students did most of the actual coding and found it helpful to work in the same room so that they could immediately coordinate their coding. Again, we remind you that defining categories for open-ended questions and the entire coding process require an enormous amount of time. At the height of their efficiency and with the codebook made up, the graduate students could each code about 10 questionnaires per hour. Coding 697 questionnaires at that rate takes a lot of time. Be sure that you budget an adequate amount of time into your planning for the analysis—especially in setting the date you indicate you will have the report ready.

Following keypunching of the data and Statistical Package for the Social Sciences (SPSS) control cards, another time-consuming activity but one that must be learned and carried out meticulously, we ran frequencies on all of the questions. We did subset comparative analyses by doing crosstabulations on all the variables by the respondents' county of residence. This enabled descriptions of each county and comparisons of all four counties on the questions asked. We also did crosstabulations of many of the questions by the respondents' age, sex, income, and marital status, since these variables are considered by many to be relatively independent ones.

The kinds and amounts of data analysis obtained from an aggregate assessment such as this one are dictated by the research questions asked, the quality of data (e.g., sample size, randomness, etc.), and the uses to which the results are to be put. Since this assessment was a descriptive baseline study using a convenience sample, our objectives were met through descriptive and comparative analyses. The entire data set or subsets can be subjected to endless secondary analyses, depending on the quality of the data and the questions one wants to ask of them. This secondary analysis can be done immediately or at a later time. For example, recent studies[5] show that older people who rate themselves as in excellent or good health live longer than people who have negative self-health ratings. We are curious to go back to the data from this 1975 and 1976 study to see if there are correlations between the respondents' ages and their self-reported health status. This kind of secondary analysis is often impossible without having the actual questionnaires available so that you can go back to the raw data.

Data from previous studies sometimes can be used for comparative analysis purposes with data from subsequent assessments. For these reasons, no matter what the storage problems are (and the space required for 697 nine-page questionnaires is considerable), we have no intention of throwing them away. To be sure, the code-books, cards, and printouts from previous analyses are valuable, but the raw data are also essential. Never throw anything away!

Uses of the assessment findings

The data from this assessment have been partially published (see the article on pp. 159-169). The major use to which the data from this assessment have been put has been for program planning and development by NDC and other agencies in their study of counties. Some of the programs that evolved as a direct result of this assess-ment include nutrition and fitness classes and increased health counseling oppor-tunities. We have also incorporated many of the findings into health education and health promotion programs. We have been able to say, "According to our study in this community, most elderly people are concerned about. . . ." The information appears to have more clout with the elderly when we are able to say that it is from people like themselves and from their own area. Obviously, some of the people in any group in the community may have actually taken part in the assessment themselves.

Other agencies and associations have also made changes in their programming as a result of the study. The Heart Association in the suburban county greatly expanded its blood pressure screening program as a result of the high level of interest in this service expressed by assessment participants. The Heart Association chapters in one of the rural counties began a blood pressure program at the senior centers and clubs in their county. A health department in one of the rural counties took the survey instrument and modified it for more extensive use in its county. Thus they have been able to build on and to expand the data base that this assessment initiated as well as to tailor those data to their specific needs and purposes.

The AAA, as primary community system participant in the assessment, also made considerable use of the assessment data in developing plans and setting priori-ties for senior services. These are activities the AAA is mandated to carry out under the Older Americans' Act. Shortly after the assessment described here was com-pleted, the AAA, with which we had worked in doing the assessment, was divided into two. One portion now serves NDC's home community. The other has jurisdic-tion over the three rural counties that were also included in the assessment. More use has been made of the data generated from the assessment in the suburban community than in the other three, partially because the preponderance of the respondents are from that county. Another reason is because NDC is active in that community and has made extensive use of the information. No large changes oc-curred immediately after the assessment except in NDC's own programming. This, although somewhat frustrating to the evaluators, is not unusual. The assessment's purpose was to provide a baseline data bank that simply had not been available before as a means of validating many of the observations providers and others working with the elderly aggregate had already made. Their findings also showed some directions for planning and service development. No dramatic changes were called for. During the period since the assessment was done and the findings were made known in the target counties, a number of services have been developed for the elderly, especially in the suburban county. It is these changes that set the stage for a second evaluation in the spring of 1981, which will be discussed in Chapter 8. For now, let us look at the questionnaire and report of the 1975 survey.

SENIOR COORDINATING COUNCIL HEALTH QUESTIONNAIRE

NOTE: IF YOU HAVE ALREADY COMPLETED THIS QUESTION-NAIRE, PLEASE *DO NOT* COMPLETE A SECOND ONE. THANK YOU!

Do not write in this space.

1. Do you come to the local senior center? ＿＿ Yes ＿＿ No
2. If yes, please check the frequency with which you attend any or all of the following activities:

Activity	Regularly	Occasionally	Never
Meals			
Crafts, e.g., oil painting			
Trips			
Recreation, e.g., folk dancing			
Cards			
Health counseling			
Social hour			
Other. Specify ＿＿＿＿＿＿＿			

3. Please check as many of the following health programs as you would like to participate in. If you have other interests, please add them at the end of the list.
   ＿＿ Cooking for 1 or 2 persons
   ＿＿ Shopping for sound nutrition
   ＿＿ Getting along with other people
   ＿＿ Posture improvement
   ＿＿ How to live with a disability
   ＿＿ Helping others live with a disability
   ＿＿ How to help local health care services better meet your needs
   ＿＿ Weight control
   ＿＿ Sex counseling
   ＿＿ Smoking control
   ＿＿ Exercise
   ＿＿ Other. Specify ＿＿＿＿＿＿＿＿＿＿＿＿＿＿＿
   ＿＿ Other. Specify ＿＿＿＿＿＿＿＿＿＿＿＿＿＿＿

Continued.

4. What kinds of exercise do you get? Check as many as apply.
_____ Walking _____ Yoga _____ Golf
_____ Gardening _____ Calisthenics _____ Tennis
_____ Housework _____ Swimming _____ Hiking
_____ Bicycling _____ Jogging _____ Bowling
_____ Regular gym or health club workouts
_____ Other. Specify _____
_____ Other. Specify _____

5. What do you do for recreation? Check as many as apply.
_____ Watch TV _____ Sew, knit, or crochet _____ Eat out
_____ Visit friends _____ Visit relatives _____ Walk
_____ Play sports _____ Play with a pet _____ Eat
_____ Sing in a choir _____ Go to church _____ Read
_____ Go to the movies _____ Play cards _____ Hike
_____ Go to the senior center _____ Go to other clubs _____ Nothing
_____ Other. Specify _____

6. What other kinds of things would you like to do?

7. Are there things you would like to do but cannot? _____ Yes _____ No
8. If yes, why can't you do them? Check as many as apply.
_____ Cannot afford
_____ No transportation
_____ Activities are not available in this area
_____ Physical limitations prevent doing them
_____ No one to do them with
_____ Other. Specify _____

9. In what type of housing do you live? Check only one.
_____ Single family home of your own
_____ Home of son or daughter
_____ Retirement complex
_____ Single room
_____ Apartment
_____ Condominium
_____ Mobile home
_____ Other. Specify _____

10. Where do you eat most of your meals? Check only one.
_____ Home
_____ Relatives' homes
_____ Senior center
_____ Friends' homes
_____ Restaurant
_____ Housing complex dining room
_____ Other. Specify _____

11. What kinds of transportation do you use? Please check all that apply.
_____ Ride with friends _____ Drive own car _____ Walk
_____ Public transit _____ Other bus _____ Taxi
_____ Senior service transportation _____ Bicycle _____ Don't get around
_____ Other. Specify _____

12. What are your biggest problems with transportation?

13. Comparing yourself with other people your age, how do you rate yourself?
Check only the *one* answer that fits best.
_____ Much better off than others
_____ Better off than others
_____ About the same as others
_____ Worse off than others
_____ Much worse off than others

14. What kind of job do you do, or did you do before retirement?

    What kind of job does or did your spouse do?

15. What kind of job did your father do?

16. From which of the following sources do you get your monthly income?
Please check as many as apply.
_____ Any kind of job
_____ Old age assistance
_____ Government pension
_____ Government payment for any kind of disability
_____ Interest from investments or rentals
_____ Savings withdrawals, sale of real estate, or cashing bonds
_____ Social Security
_____ Private pension
_____ Relatives
_____ Other. Specify _____

17. Which one of the following categories most closely approximates your
monthly income? Please check only one.
_____ None
_____ Less than $300
_____ $300 to $499
_____ $500 to $999
_____ $1,000 to $1,499
_____ $1,500 to $1,999
_____ $2,000 to $2,499
_____ $2,500 or more

18. What do you consider your home state? _____
19. In what town do you live now? _____
20. How long have you lived where you are living now? Check only one.
_____ Under a year
_____ More than 1 year but less than 2 years
_____ More than 2 years but less than 5 years
_____ Five years or longer

21. Do you attend religious services? _____ Yes _____ No
22. If yes, would you give us some of the reasons you go to religious services;
for example: religion is personally meaningful; going to services provides
socializing opportunities, etc.

Continued.

SENIOR COORDINATING COUNCIL HEALTH QUESTIONNAIRE—cont'd

23. What's the one best thing about your life now?

Do not
write
in this
space.

24. What's the one worst thing about your life now?

25. Please give us your birth date. _____
                                   month   day   year
26. What is your sex? ____ Male   ____ Female
27. What is your marital status? Please check only one.
    ____ Married   ____ Divorced ____ Widowed ____ Single
    ____ Separated ____ Spouse hospitalized or in nursing home
28. With whom do you live? ____ Spouse ____ Alone
    ____ Son or daughter ____ Friend ____ Other relative
    ____ Other. Who? _____
29. Do you have someone in whom you can confide and talk over personal
    problems? ____ Yes   ____ No
30. If yes, what relationship is this person to you? Please check as many as
    apply.
    ____ Spouse   ____ Friend ____ Nurse   ____ Physician
    ____ Daughter or son ____ Neighbor ____ Clergyman
    ____ Brother or sister ____ Social worker ____ Other.
    Specify _____
31. The following is a list of conditions often experienced by older persons.
    Please check any of these conditions which you have been told by a doctor
    that you have or that *you* think you have.

Condition	Doctor told you you have	You think you have
Arthritis	____	____
Cancer. What organ?	____	____
Cataract	____	____
Diabetes	____	____
Emphysema	____	____
Glaucoma	____	____
Gout	____	____
Heart attack	____	____
Hiatus hernia	____	____
High blood pressure	____	____
Kidney disease/stones	____	____
Loss of hearing	____	____
Rheumatic heart trouble	____	____
Shortness of breath	____	____
Stroke	____	____
Stomach ulcer	____	____
Thyroid disease	____	____
Other. Specify _____		

Do not
write
in this
space.

32. Do you smoke? _____ Yes _____ No
    If yes, how much per day? _____

33. In a day, how many cups do you drink of _____ tea _____ coffee
    _____ cola?

34. Do you drink decaffeinated coffee? _____ Yes _____ No

35. How many alcohol drinks do you have a day? _____

36. Is your activity limited in any way by a physical disability?
    _____ Yes _____ No
    If yes, please specify what kind of disability limits your activity.
    _____

37. Do you have your own physician? _____ Yes _____ No

38. How many months has it been since you last saw a physician?
    _____ months

39. Why did you go to a physician the last time you went?
    _____ Regular physical examination _____ Illness
    What kind of illness? _____
    Other. Specify _____

40. How many times in the past 12 months have you *not* gone to a physician
    when you thought you should go? _____ times

41. If you did not go to a physician when you thought you should, what kept
    you from going? Please check as many as apply.
    _____ Lack of transportation   _____ Have no doctor
    _____ Could not get an appointment   _____ Too busy to go
    _____ Could not afford to go to a doctor
    _____ Doctor doesn't listen to you
    _____ Other. Specify _____

42. Have you been hospitalized during the last 12 months?
    _____ Yes _____ No

43. If yes, for what were you hospitalized? Please be specific.
    _____

44. How many months has it been since you had a protoscopic (rectal) exami-
    nation? _____ months.

45. Women: How many months has it been since you had a pelvic examination
    which included a Pap test for cancer of the cervix? _____ months.

46. Women: Do you examine your own breasts regularly once a month for
    lumps? _____ Yes _____ No

47. Please tell us what kinds of health insurance coverage you have; e.g.,
    Medicare, Retired Teachers, Etna, etc. Please list all companies.

48. Have you used your health insurance? _____ Yes _____ No

49. Are you satisfied with your health insurance coverage?
    _____ Yes _____ No

50. If no, please tell us why you are not satisfied with your health insurance.

Continued.

SENIOR COORDINATING COUNCIL HEALTH QUESTIONNAIRE—cont'd

51. Please list the name and dosage of all medicines which you take. Also please tell us how often you take them and for what. Include prescriptions, laxatives, vitamins, diet supplements, stomach pills, sleeping pills, aspirin, etc.

Do not write in this space.

Medicine	Dosage	How often	For what

52. The words in the list below describe some of the ways people feel about themselves and about life. Please put a check mark on the line after each of the words which best indicates how much or how often the word described the way you think or feel. For example, if you are generally a happy person, you would put a check mark on the "very often" line after happy.

Choices

Words	Never	Very rarely	Rarely	Sometimes	Very often	Always
Angry	___	___	___	___	___	___
Bored	___	___	___	___	___	___
Depressed	___	___	___	___	___	___
Frightened	___	___	___	___	___	___
Happy	___	___	___	___	___	___
Lonely	___	___	___	___	___	___
Overwhelmed	___	___	___	___	___	___
Satisfied	___	___	___	___	___	___
Secure	___	___	___	___	___	___
Other. List						

**THANK YOU FOR YOUR HELP AND COOPERATION
IN COMPLETING THIS QUESTIONNAIRE.**

LIFE-STYLE INDICATORS FOR INTERVENTIONS TO
FACILITATE ELDERLY PERSONS' INDEPENDENCE*

Sarah Ellen Archer, RN, Dr.PH
Ruth P. Fleshman, RN, MS
Carol L. Carver, RN, MS
Lannie Adelman, RN, MS

Mrs. Tucci beams as she reads her weight on the scale; she has lost three more pounds as a result of our "Remodeling Yourself" class. At 70, she looks no more than 60; more importantly, she says she feels better than she has in years. She's more limber now and can walk more easily in spite of her bad knee. Mr. Thomas, who used to salt all his food before he had even tasted it, tells about complaining to the waiter last night because his entrée was oversalted. He's walking more, bowling twice a week, and his blood pressure is down to 150/92 without medication. He says he's beginning to enjoy retirement. These anecdotes may represent small changes in the big picture of overall health care in the United States, but the impact on the lives of these elderly clients is great.

Our objective for working with elderly people in the community is to help them maintain their independence and optimal level of functioning.[1] Toward this end, we have situated our practice[2] in senior centers, Title VII dining sites and senior clubs—places where community elderly people come and where we can be accessible to them. Our primary focus is on helping clients adapt current health information into forms which they can utilize with as little disruption of their total life-style as possible. In addition, we do health maintenance counseling, selected screening and referrals to other health and medical resources. These activities have enabled us to become an available and nonthreatening source of health information and assistance for our clients as well as other professionals and groups who work with them. A continual reward for us is feedback from clients about how useful our information and services are to them. A common comment is, "finally, I've found someone who will listen to me and answer my questions so I can understand."

Our current work with older adults evolved from a request for us to develop a blood pressure monitoring service at the largest local senior center. The request

*From Health Values: achieving high level wellness 3(3), Thorofare, N.J., 1979, Charles B. Slack, Inc.

This study was supported by Nursing Dynamics Corporation, Mill Valley, California, and funds from the Biomedical Research Support Grant RR 05604-04 awarded by the Biomedical Research Support Program. Division of Research Resources, National Institutes of Health, to the School of Nursing. University of California, San Francisco.

Adapted from a speech presented at the American Public Health Association, Annual Meeting, Washington, D.C., November 1977.

Requests for reprints should be addressed to Sarah Ellen Archer, RN, Dr.Ph. School of Nursing, Department of Mental Health and Community Nursing, University of California, Room N505-Y, San Francisco, California 94143.

came as a result of an experimental program for health education and blood pressure screening we conducted in a community pharmacy in 1974.[3] We have made it clear from the outset in all of our work with older adults that we were committed to primary prevention and health promotion first, and would use blood pressure monitoring and other screening procedures as means to draw people into the health education and health counseling program.

After a few months of work with the clients and much searching through local data sources such as comprehensive health planning, area agencies on aging, county and city planning departments and other organizations working with older adults, we realized that baseline data on the needs, wants and life-styles of our clients were sorely lacking. Needs assessments had been done, to be sure, but they were by and large based on the educated guesses of various local service providers. No systematically gathered data from community elderly people *themselves* were available. We needed these data to use as a basis for planning health classes and services based on *their* own priorities. Of course, we had considerable case data on individuals, which were very useful in planning for them. Because of our preparation as community health nurses, we were well aware of the impact on other programs' planners of epidemiological data on the population of elderly people living in the communities in which we were working. Since these data were not available, we set out to collect them. The study's findings and their later uses presented here are what we feel are of most interest to other health practitioners working in community settings with the objectives of primary prevention and health promotion.

Study methodology

Because our target population is a socially active one, utilizing senior centers, clubs and Title VII dining sites, we chose these sites for the conduct of our survey. We began with our own suburban northern California county, and were soon invited to expand the study into three adjacent rural counties. This would enable us and other agencies to have baseline data for each of the four counties as well as opportunities to make comparisons among them. This expansion was particularly appropriate since all four study counties were under the aegis of the same Area Agency on Aging, which was charged with developing comprehensive plans for meeting the needs of elderly residents.

Entry into community agencies as well as to individuals for study is an increasingly difficult aspect of conducting survey research. Many people, especially the elderly, feel that they have been overstudied.[4] So they are becoming resistive to filling out questionnaires, especially from strangers or groups from whom the return for them personally is unknown or nonexistent. Knowing these phenomena, we set out to gain access to groups of community elderly through the people who coordinated the senior centers, clubs and dining sites. Because we were well known in our own county through our work with both the older adults and those who worked with them, we had relatively easy access to groups. Our presentations had to wait, however, until their agendas permitted time for us to be scheduled to come and conduct the study during regular meetings or activities. In the other three counties we had to depend greatly on the introductions and endorsement from the Area Agency on Aging to obtain permission to visit study sites. Some of the coordinators in the other three counties proved to be very effective gatekeepers, and we were unable to obtain data from their activities' participants. As is the case with many studies of this kind, we ended up with a convenient sample of sites to which we could gain access.

In many instances we were permitted to present a part of the program meeting or after-luncheon or dinner activities on health, as well as given the opportunity to invite those in attendance to participate in the study, by completing our questionnaire. We were delighted to do this since it gave us a chance to share information as well as to provide some tangible service for the participants in return for their time to fill out the questionnaire. Such presentations also aided the research project, since we were able to demonstrate to the audience that we were helpful people whose research would be harmless to them as participants. We administered the anonymous questionnaire to all who volunteered to complete it, and gave instructions to and answered questions from the group as a whole. We found that our returns were much better if we remained on the scene and collected the questionnaires ourselves rather than relying on the coordinators or individual participants to get them back to us. Our efforts between May 1975 and May 1976 netted 679 questionnaires on which usable data were provided.

Findings and discussion

Demographic data. Six-hundred and thirty of the 679 respondents indicated their sex.* Of these, 79% were female and 21% male. The median age was 69.3 years, mean age was 69.5 years and modal age was in the 70 to 74 age group. Forty-two percent were married, 45% widowed, 7% single, 5% divorced and the other 1% were separated either voluntarily or through institutionalization of the spouse. Forty-eight percent live alone, 40% with their spouse, 6% with a son or daughter, 4% with another relative and 2% with a friend. In response to the question about how long they had lived where they are living now, 68% indicate five years or longer, 17% between two and five years and 14% less than two years. Eighty-nine percent lived in a single-family unit such as a house, apartment, condominium or mobile home, 5% lived with a son, daughter or other relative, 5% in a retirement or low cost housing complex and less than 1% in a single room. Modal income was between $500 and $999 a month, median income was $400 a month and mean income $440. More than 98% of the respondents were Caucasian.

---

*All percentages are based on the number of respondents answering the questions, which in many instances is less than 679.

Life-style indicators. Recreation is essential to enable people to have a change of pace, cope with stress and recharge their physical, psychological and emotional batteries. Ambulatory elderly respondents were asked what they did for recreation. The array of activities was combined into the six types of recreation shown in Table I. Sedentary recreational activities indicated by 94% of the respondents included watching TV, sewing, playing cards, eating and reading. With the exception of playing cards, these behaviors, along with playing with a pet, were classified as isolate behaviors. Playing cards, visiting friends and relatives and dancing were considered to be social forms of recreation because of their direct involvement with other people. Eighty-seven percent of the respondents indicated participation in social recreation because of their direct involvement with other people. Semisocial recreational activities were so designated because they involve leaving the individual's home, but do not require direct interaction with other people as do the activities classed as social. Semisocial recreational activities included attending church, eating out, going to the movies, singing in a choir, traveling, working, playing sports and attending a senior center or senior club. Less than half of the respondents indicated active types of recreation such as hiking, playing sports, walking or dancing. Only 3% indicated no recreational activities at all.

The type of exercise people get is being increasingly recognized as an influencing factor on cardiovascular functioning as well as health status in general. Table II contains respondents' reporting of the kinds of exercise they get. Ninety-eight percent reported light exercise. Activities included in light exercise were walking, gardening, housework, yoga and bowling. Strenuous exercise in this study referred to calisthenics, swimming, jogging, tennis and hiking. Twenty-three percent of the respondents indicated they did such activities. Fifteen percent participated in moderate exercise, which included bicycling, health club or spa, golf, dancing and climbing stairs. Five participants, or less than 1%, indicated they got no exercise at all.

Mobility in the American society is essential, particularly in geographical areas such as the target counties where distances are great and public transportation leaves much to be desired. Driving one's own car continues to be the leading mode of transportation. Thirty-four percent walk and 33% ride the bus. Only 6% indicated use of taxis. In response to the question of whether there were activities respondents would like to do but could not, 71% answered yes. Only 129 cited reasons for their answer. Thirty-eight percent could not afford to do what they wanted to, 37% were impeded by physical limitations, 35% had no transportation, 27% had no one with whom to do the desired activities and 18% reported that the activities they wanted were not available in the area. Less than 1% each reported that they were afraid to go out, were new to the area or had no time for other activities.

Participants were asked to rank themselves compared to other people their own age. Twenty-one percent indicated that they were much better off than others their age, 30% better off and 34% felt they were about the same as others. Less than 2%

TABLE I

Types of recreation reported by ambulatory elderly participants (n = 663)

Type of recreation	Number of participants reporting	Percent of participants
Sedentary	618	94
Active	322	49
Isolate	617	93
Semisocial	553	84
Social	572	87
None	18	3

TABLE II

Types of exercise reported by ambulatory elderly participants (n = 638)

Type of exercise	Number of participants reporting*	Percent of participants
Strenuous	146	23
Moderate	97	15
Light	625	98
None	5	1

*Many participants reported more than one type of exercise.

ranked themselves as worse off than others. This very high ranking of selves compared to others may be reflective of the fact that our respondents were all active members of their community and may have been comparing themselves to the stereotypes often applied to the elderly: sick, alone, poor and institutionalized. Certainly our respondents do not fit these stereotypes.

Respondents were asked in open-ended questions to tell us what was the "best" and what was the "worst" thing about their lives at the time they answered the question. These were apparently difficult questions for the participants to answer, since only 189 gave information about best and 101 gave information about worst aspects of life. The most frequently given best thing was health, which was listed by 54 (28%) of the respondents. Other best aspects of life shown in Table III included family, leisure time, retirement, friends and social life and senior clubs and activities. Health problems, including unspecified disabilities, cataracts, arthritis, failing eyesight, alcoholism, nervousness, loss of memory and tension, led the list of factors which respondents identified as "worst" in their lives (Table IV). All of these health problems interfere with the person's abilities to function and bring them potentially closer to what so many older people have told us they fear more than death—

TABLE III

Respondents' identification of one best thing in their lives (n = 189)

Best thing	Number of participants reporting	Percent of participants
Health	54	28
Family	37	20
Leisure/free time	29	15
Retirement/no work	19	10
Friends/social life	14	8
Senior clubs and activities	7	5
General happiness	6	3
Keeping busy/useful	6	3
Financial independence	5	3
Home/place where live	4	2
Other*	6	3
Total	189	100

*Includes religion, coping with widowhood, using the past and travel.

TABLE IV

Respondents' identification of one worst thing in their lives (n = 101)

Worst thing	Number of participants reporting	Percent of participants
Health problems	26	26
Loneliness	20	20
Death of husband	7	7
Inflation and taxes	7	7
Illness: spouse, family, friends	7	7
Not enough time	6	6
Old age	6	6
Transportation problems	6	6
Lack of money	5	5
Boredom	3	3
House and garden work	2	1
Other*	6	6
Total	101	100

*Includes fear of crime, sorry for unsaved people, government and moral breakdown, live far from family, husband around and bossy, living on a hill.

disability producing dependence. Loneliness ranks second, and can be assumed to be related to other factors listed such as death of the husband and illness of spouse, family and friends, as well as to transportation and financial problems. Factors listed under old age included loss of strength and inability to do what the person could do at age 40. The margin by which health leads both the lists of best and worst factors in their lives underscores older persons' realization of the importance of their health in their total lives.

Respondents were presented a list of words which described selected emotions such as happy, frightened, secure and lonely. They were asked to rank themselves in the category on a Likert Scale which best described how they thought or felt relative to each named emotion. The rankings in percentage of participants responding to each of the selected emotions are presented in Table V. It is interesting to note that the numbers of respondents ranking themselves varies with each of the emotions given; the range of numbers of respondents is from a high of 465 for "happy" to a low of 248 for "overwhelmed." Some respondents did not understand the meaning of "overwhelmed," and that may account for the low number of people ranking themselves on that emotion. Three of the nine emotions given—"happy," "satisfied" and "secure"—have positive valence, while the other six are negative. These three positive-valence emotions received three of the four highest numerical responses from participants. "Angry," which may actually be a positive-valence emotion, received the third highest response rate. The positive aspects of anger may lie in the possibility that its expression indicates active and personal rejection of the sterotypical role of the aged which many of the elderly are discovering is not as bad as they had been led

TABLE V

Elderly respondents' rankings of the frequency or extent to which they experience selected emotions

Selected emotions	Percent of respondents indicating each choice						Number ranking themselves on each word
	Never	Very rarely	Rarely	Sometimes	Very often	Always	
Angry	5	34	21	36	4	1	360
Bored	23	22	17	32	6	1	333
Depressed	17	22	14	42	5	1	335
Frightened	34	23	14	23	5	1	310
Happy	6	1	2	12	59	21	465
Lonely	27	17	14	32	8	1	338
Overwhelmed	31	16	17	26	6	4	249
Satisfied	6	1	1	15	55	23	379
Secure	5	1	3	12	42	37	347

to believe it would be. This possibility seems to be supported by the respondents' rankings of themselves compared to others as it may also be by their high response rates on "happy," "secure" and "satisfied." The relatively low rate of responses to "frightened" can be attributed in great measure to the fact that the geographical areas where respondents live are suburban and rural. A much higher response to this emotion could be anticipated from urban and particularly elderly inner city dwellers.

The higher responses on positive-valence emotions indicate that the elderly, like the rest of us, are more comfortable expressing positive or acceptable emotions and feelings than in sharing more negative ones. This finding is supported by the fact that, as noted above, 189 respondents expressed what was best about their lives, but only 101 were willing to indicate what was worst. Those of us who work with older adults might be well advised to bear in mind this apparent tendency, and so approach our older clients with a "what's good about your life" perspective as well as a "problem-oriented" one.

Activities respondents would like. As a direct aid to senior center and senior club staff, as well as to ourselves and to other service providers, participants were asked what health promotional programs they would like through centers and clubs. Their anwers are given in Table VI. Weight control was their number one request, with exercise classes a fairly close second. Other related requests for health promotional programs were cooking for one or two persons, shopping for sound nutrition and posture improvement. Almost one third of the respondents wanted assistance in helping health care services to better meet their demands. Only 8% wanted assistance with smoking control.

TABLE VI

Health promotional programs ambulatory elderly participants would like through their senior centers and senior clubs

Health promotional program	Number of participants responding*	Percent of participants responding
Weight control	195	45
Exercise	173	40
Cooking for 1 or 2 persons	157	36
Blood pressure checks	134	31
Shopping for sound nutrition	109	25
Getting along with other people	93	21
Posture improvement	92	21
How to live with a disability	80	18
Helping others live with a disability	76	17
How to help local health care services better	71	16
Smoking control	35	8
Sex counseling	21	5

*Many participants desired more than one health promotional program.

Uses to which the survey findings have been put

One of the greatest challenges we have faced in developing health promotional services for well older people in their own communities has been the constant admonition that we should instead be focusing on severely handicapped and/or hard-to-reach elderly as the County Health Department was planning to do. Others have counseled that we should be concentrating our efforts on school-age children and young people where potential long-term payoff is great. When we approached the local Adult Education Department to help us develop classes for the elderly in clubs and centers, the personnel at Adult Ed wanted us to begin our classes in nursing homes where so many elderly people were in need of them. The staff was startled to learn that at any given point, 95% of all elderly people are living in the community and only 5% are in institutions.[5] We have stressed to all of these colleagues that our objective is to increase services for community elderly to help them maintain their optimal level of functioning in order to at least postpone, if not totally prevent, disability and loss of independence. We have continued to demonstrate the need for such activities, ways to implement them and some of the results which can be expected from them. In so doing we have filled gaps in existing services and have served as role models for other providers. The epidemiological data partially reported here as well as our individual case histories have given us a broad data base as a guide for our own activities through Nursing Dynamics Corporation as well as information to share with other agencies.

The first thing we did on the basis of the study findings was to organize a series of "Remodeling Yourself" classes, which addresses our clients' stated desires for information and instruction on weight control, exercise, cooking, shopping for sound nutrition and posture improvement (Table VI). The class has a three-pronged approach: exercise, nutrition and relaxation. We have arranged for the classes to be sponsored by Adult Education, so that they became involved with well elderly and to enable the nurse and dietitian team of instructors to be paid for their teaching. These Remodeling Yourself classes have been going on since mid-1976, and continue to be popular with our clientele. We also refer many of our own clients who are overweight, tense and who have elevated blood pressures to these classes.

Throughout the study period and since, we have applied many of the findings into our own practice of health counseling and promotion. More emphasis in both history taking and health education is placed on diet, recreation, exercise, tobacco, caffeine and alcohol usage and the recency of specific diagnostic examinations. We have also shared the findings with graduate nursing and pharmacy students who have done field work with us.

We have given reports of the study findings to local planning and provider agencies. The data have been used in developing area plans by the Area Agencies on Aging responsible for the counties where the study was conducted. They have served as a basis for inservice programs on life-style characteristics of their clientele for providers of services to community elderly. The findings have helped justify expanded services by local official and voluntary agencies. For example, as a result of respondents' stated desire for blood pressure checks in senior centers and clubs, Nursing Dynamics Corporation has expanded our services into other centers, clubs and dining sites; the Heart Association extended its screening program; and at least one of the other county's health departments has begun to offer blood pressure screening at senior centers and dining sites in their jurisdiction. Another county's health department has modified our original questionnaire and is using it for an extensive survey of areas of their county which we were unable to reach. Their data, combined with what Nursing Dynamics has given them, have provided them with a baseline data bank.

The so-called health care system is often accused of failure to address problems of the aged before they reach the level of rank pathology, and nowhere have we found this more true than in the mental health agencies. In spite of our findings reporting the interrelated concerns and joys of old age (Tables III and IV), and extensive research demonstrating the increased vulnerability to the total health of the aged from assaults on any aspect of life,[5,6] the community mental health services seem only theoretically aware of a prevention approach to health. Local providers have been interest in our findings; our data were incorporated into the annual plan for mental health services. However, they have done little to modify their services, dealing instead with drug-abusing youth and child-abusing families. As a result, we have had to increase our own emphasis on mental health aspects of our practice, and have sought consultation from other nurses, more skilled at mental health interventions than we are, to help our elderly clients. We have encouraged one aged community resident in her founding and running of a support group for other women who, like herself, have been caring for husbands severely disabled from strokes. Because we have gotten nowhere with community mental health centers, we have turned to family service agencies to establish widows' groups and other mental health services for community elderly.

It is very difficult to assess the effects of sharing our findings on individual and group care providers. Through our participation in a variety of community service activities with other providers, we have been able to make many of them aware of what we have found and some of the things we think need to be done as a result. One of us teaches in a school of nursing and has made use of the study's methodology and its findings with several classes of graduate students. In addition, a series of classes through the local university extension's continuing education program is planned to make a systematic effort to reach nurses who are already working with older people.

Conclusion

The study reported here is an example of the role survey research can play in the development and use of a data base for program planning and implementation.

Although individual providers often have a wealth of case-by-case anecdotes, extrapolations made from these data to entire populations are of questionable validity as a sole basis for planning services. Survey methodology provides opportunity to systematically gather epidemiologic data from large numbers of people in many community settings. This outreach into the community carries with it the potential for reaching people who may not otherwise be known to the system. This study did just that. Its results highlight, for the researcher and others in the target area, the reality of the high level of functioning many elderly people enjoy and want to maintain. They further rout the myth that old equals sick.

References

1. Archer SE, Fleshman, RP: Community Health Nursing: Patterns and Practice. North Scituate, Massachusetts, Duxbury Press, 1975
2. Archer SE, Fleshman RP: Doing our own thing: Community health nurses in independent practice. J Nurs Admin, in press.
3. Fleshman RP, Archer SE: Nurse-pharmacist teams screen for hypertension. Hosp Formulary 11:73-81, 1976.
4. Bulbul PI: Everybody's Studying Us: The Ironies of Aging in the Pepsi Generation. San Francisco, Glide Publications, 1976.
5. Shanas E et al: Old People in Three Industrial Societies. New York, Atherton Press, 1968.
6. Butler RN, Lewis MI: Aging and Mental Health. St. Louis, CV Mosby Co. 1973.
7. Youmans EG, Yarrow M: Aging and social adaptation: A longitudinal study of healthy old men.

In Branick S, Patterson RD (eds.): Human Aging II: An Eleven Year Follow-up Biomedical and Behavioral Study. Besthesda, Maryland, USDHEW Pub No. 71-9037, 1971.

Bibliography

Binstock RH, Shanas E (eds): Handbook of Aging and the Social Sciences. New York, Van Nostrand Reinhold Co, 1976.
Birren JE et al: Human Aging. Bethesda, Maryland, USDHEW Pub No. 986, 1963.
Butler RN: Why Survive? Being Old in America. New York, Harper & Row, 1975.
Lowenthal MF: Lives in Distress. New York, Basic Books, 1964.
Neugarten BL (ed): Middle Age and Aging. Chicago, University of Chicago Press, 1968.
Palmore E (ed): Normal Aging. Durham, North Carolina, Duke University Press, 1970.

REFERENCES TO CHAPTER 7

1. Archer, S.E., and Fleshman, R.P.: Doing our own thing: community health nurses in indepedent practice, Journal of Nursing Administration 8:44-51, November 1978.
2. Archer, S.E., and Fleshman, R.P.: Community Health Nursing: patterns and practice, North Scituate, Mass., 1979, Duxbury Press.
3. Archer, S.E., and Fleshman, R.P.: Faculty role modeling: opportunities presented by Nursing Dynamics Corporation, Nursing Outlook 29:586-589, October 1981.
4. Nie, N.H., and others: Statistical package for the social sciences, ed. 2, New York, 1975, McGraw-Hill Book Co.
5. Mossey, J.M., and Shapiro, E.: Self-related health: a predictor of mortality among the elderly, American Journal of Public Health 72:800-808, August 1982.

8

SENIOR RESOURCES SURVEY

OVERVIEW

Carole Kelly and Sarah Archer conducted this evaluation for a variety of reasons. At the time Sarah Archer was an officer on the advisory Commission on Aging for the AAA and chair of its Health Committee. The AAA, as part of its charge to develop and implement an annual plan as well as long-range plans for the elderly in its community, needed information about senior citizens' knowledge and potential use of the services that already existed for them. In addition, the AAA wanted to ask some questions about older residents' retirement experiences and their planning for possible future illness. Nursing Dynamics Corporation (NDC) had amassed considerable information about and experience with seniors and senior services in the county. At the same time we were in the process of developing a new undergraduate community assessment course in the school of nursing. We planned to offer this course in conjunction with the graduate community health nursing course in community organization. We decided to use these courses as the vehicle for meeting the AAA's needs for an aggregate assessment and to use the community as the site for the clinical experience in both courses. The collaborative intersystem for this evaluation was composed of the AAA's program manager and planner from the community system and us as representatives of the consultant system. This evaluation was conducted under a formal consultation contract.

Consultative evaluation intersystem members met several times with the staff members from the AAA to develop the design and schedule for the evaluation. In addition to the AAA's frame, we also had to cope with the university's quarter-system calendar. The contract with the AAA for the evaluation was from September 1980 to August 1981. Again we found that everyone wanted a number of favorite questions included on the evaluation tool. We had to pare it down several times to keep it a manageable length. We had learned the pitfalls of a long questionnaire all too well from our first experience with assessing the elderly aggregate in this community.

Although the AAA wanted the evaluation, it had no funds to pay for the project nor did NDC. Since the assessment was a project in required community health nursing courses at the undergraduate and graduate levels, we sought and obtained funds from the University of California-San Francisco School of Nursing to appoint graduate student teaching assistants to help in the development and conduct of the undergraduate course, which would have 39 students in it. The university again supplied computer support, since the project was a research learning experience for the graduate students. The undergraduate students did the actual interviewing of volunteer respondents as their field work in the course; the graduate students supervised teams of undergraduates and actively participated in the coding and the computer analysis of the data. The process followed the learn-by-doing and faculty role-modeling approach that has worked so well in the past.[1]

We submitted the report to the AAA in the fall of 1981, missing our original deadline by 2 months. In retrospect, considering the number of obstacles in the process and the challenges of having some 55 students involved, we are relieved that the report was no later than that.

Evaluation design

As had been the case with our first assessment of the elderly in our target county, we used a descriptive cross-sectional design. Once again the Social Security lists were not available, so we could not sample potential respondents on a random basis. After lengthy discussion with our colleagues at the AAA, we decided that seeking respondents at senior centers, clubs, and dining sites was inappropriate for this study since the respondents obtained in this way would bias the study by overrepresenting people who were already a part of many of the senior services. We therefore had to come up with another approach to try to get a greater cross-section of the target population to volunteer to participate. We finally decided to try the media (see Fig. 4, p. 76).

We sent announcements stating the purpose of the evaluation and details of its conduct to all kinds of media within the county. Both the general press and the newsletters and other publications directed specifically at seniors were very cooperative. The announcements invited interested seniors to volunteer to be interviewed by calling one of the local information and referral services to leave their name, address, and phone number. An interviewer would then contact each volunteer to arrange a mutually convenient time and place for the interview.

Because of a variety of circumstances beyond our control, fewer elderly people than we had expected actually volunteered. Somehow researchers tend to believe that potential respondents will be as interested in the research as we are and so will rush to volunteer. However, this is not usually the case. The most problematic of these uncontrollable circumstances was that several other surveys of the elderly population were already in progress. The people, justifiably, apparently thought that they were being overstudied at that time.

Since we had already considered the contingency of too few volunteers from the first advertisement, we advertised again. This second media blitz did not generate enough volunteers either. We were going to have to find other ways of gaining access to them, so we went to our final alternative, to seek out potential respondents at dining sites, blood pressure clinics, and congregate housing sites. We still believed that these three sites would provide a more representative group of elderly that we could contact if we returned to the clubs and centers. In the end we successfully interviewed 138 people. Approximately half of these respondents entered the study through volunteer response to the media invitation; we initiated contact with the others from referrals given us from dining, blood pressure, or congregate housing sites in the community.

All subjects were self-selected, which serves as a source of bias in the samples (see Chapter 5). It is possible that the people who responded to the media and congregate site invitations to participate in the study were people who are more aware of and more likely to participate in services for older people than were nonvolunteers. Thus the bias resulting from an all-volunteer sample is likely to be in the direction of interviewing people who know more about services and are more rather than less involved in them.

Because the rural western part of the county had recently been the scene of a door-to-door needs assessment of the elderly resident population by a local senior services agency, we purposely did not seek out volunteers for this assessment from that area. Instead we made questions on our instrument as comparable as possible to those in this earlier study. In this way we sought to have at least some data on both surveys that could be compared.

The overall time line for the evaluation is shown in Fig. 7 (see also Fig. 2, p. 32). The contract with the AAA was finalized in September 1980. Instrument development and pretesting were done during the university's fall quarter. During the winter quarter, 1981, we developed the community health nursing courses in which the evaluation would be conducted. We also worked with the AAA staff and representatives from other agencies to prepare the media anouncements for release in March. By late March it was obvious that we were not going to receive the number of volunteers we had hoped to reach through the media and so the contingency plans were activated. Thus we spent a great deal of time in late March and early April seeking out volunteers through dining sites, blood pressure programs, and congregate housing. The community health nursing courses were offered in the spring quarters, and students did all of the interviews in April and May.

The graduate students, under Sally Bisch's guidance, began data analysis in May. Completion of the analysis was coordinated by one of the master's students, Meladee Stankus. This phase took longer than we had planned. Carole Kelly and Sarah Archer completed the final report in September and Carole Kelly presented it to the AAA in

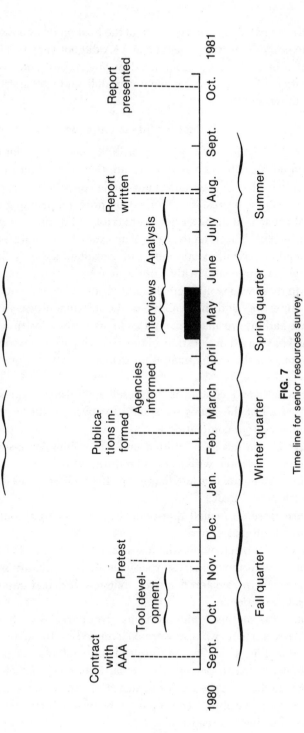

FIG. 7
Time line for senior resources survey.

October 1981. As noted, the presentation of the final report was 3 months beyond our original time frame. Our colleagues at the AAA did not view this fact with particular concern, since limited work is conducted during August and even September because of vacations. Vacations also make it very difficult to get assistance and consultation during those months.

Instrument construction

Carole Kelly assumed primary responsibility for instrument development. She worked continuously with AAA staff to be sure that content they believed was essential was included. She used the interview guide construction as part of her work in Sarah Archer's course on research methods in program planning and evaluation. As such, several versions of the interview were critiqued during the course by members of the graduate class. This is an example of an evaluator seeking feedback and validation from members of both community and consultant systems. The final version of the interview was pretested with elderly members of the community who were comparable to those who would actually participate in the evaluation. Revisions were made after pretesting, and thus validity of the instrument was increased.

As noted earlier, we made many questions on our instrument comparable to those that had been used in the study of the western part of the county. We chose the interview format for this evaluation rather than a self-administered questionnaire for several reasons:

1. The length and complexity of a self-administered questionnaire that addressed all of the issues we sought to cover would have discouraged most volunteers from completing it.
2. The interview format permitted uniform probing for answers that would not have been possible with a self-administered tool.
3. A questionnaire of this length (see pp. 194-205) would have been expensive to reproduce and mail.
4. Return rates on mailed questionnaires are generally much lower than are returns from interviews.
5. One of the objectives for the assessment was to provide the undergraduate students with interviewing experience in a community setting. All of these students were registered nurses, but few had had any community health nursing experience.
6. Timing was another important factor. Not only did we have a schedule from the AAA to meet, we also were constrained by the university's quarter system (see Fig. 4, p. 76). We wanted the students not only to have an opportunity to participate in the actual interviews but also to have at least initial feedback on the results so that they could have a feeling of the project completion. We also placed copies of the final report in the learning resources center for them to read.

Needless to say, we did not accomplish everything we set out to do. In one instance we left out a "not applicable" response (question 33). As a result we were only able to list responses in the analysis instead of being able to do some comparisons. The other problem we encountered was a lack of understanding by some of the students. In spite of the training and the practice that the students had, there was some confusion over the first section of the questionnaire (questions 1 and 2). The students were to record the responses on an answer sheet (see pp. 192-193). If a respondent gave a negative answer about knowledge of a specific service, the student was to go to the next service. If one does not know about a service, one cannot answer questions about her or his own use or others' use of that service. Those answer sheets that had responses after an initial negative response were discarded. This reduced our number of respondents from 156 to 138.

Question 2 dealt with mental health services. Only 115 of those questioned gave a response. This is a sensitive area for the elderly. For many, it is not a socially accepted service. The format of the question added to the confusion for a few students and limited the number of accurately recorded responses.

As we stated regarding the first study, the desire to include everything in a survey is an overwhelming one. In addition, the desire of the client agency to take advantage of an opportunity to get much needed data at no cost was also great. We also wanted to expose the students to a real-life experience rather then an academic exercise. All these factors together led to a survey that was much too long and too broad. The good points, however, were that it really laid some groundwork for future studies, it exposed the students to the realities of trying to gather information in the real world, and it made us all aware of how long it takes to complete such an effort. We did have the complete support of the AAA and were very appreciative of the fact that they did not pressure us to complete our work. The whole process strengthened relationships between the university and the AAA.

Preparing investigators

Investigator preparation was a major undertaking, especially with regard to working with the undergraduate students, since the interviews were the major portion of their field experience for the community health nursing course on community assessment. Lectures were devoted to didactic content about community and aggregate assessment. Seminars and field work were concerned with the process of the actual evaluation. Ruth Fleshman, president of NDC, conducted 6 hours of interviewer preparation (see pp. 183-194). She was able to give the students a great deal of information about the community and the target elderly aggregate, as well as to supervise their role-playing sessions with the interview guide. We provided several supervised practice interview sessions so that the undergraduate students were thoroughly familiar with the instrument and with the use of uniform probing questions. Through this preparation we sought to ensure interview uniformity to increase reliability. This is a very important consideration because we had 39 interviewers. The large number of interviewers, despite extensive preparation, is a limitation of this evaluation.

We also presented each student with an extensive training module based on Babbie's survey research work.[2] In addition, interviewer dress and grooming were topics of these sessions. Appropriate dress for students on campus is often not appropriate when they are representing community agencies and the university in interviewer situations. Thus the interviewer preparation sessions covered more than just the conduct of the interviews. As another means of assuring reliability of the data, master's level students supervised teams of undergraduate student interviewers, went over completed interviews, and discussed discrepancies or missing information with the individual interviewer as soon as possible. Sally Bisch, a doctoral student in the course, took major responsibility for working with the master's students in data analysis. All of the graduate students met in separate seminars to discuss course content, interviewing experiences with the undergraduate students, and data analysis techniques and results. Carole Kelly and Nancy Schwartz, the two teaching assistants, were active throughout the process and carried major responsibilities for the survey as well as for teaching some of the classes. At times things went very well, at other times it was chaotic. Sarah Archer had to oversee it all.

Informed consent

We followed the university's Human Research Committee's procedure for review of all research projects involving human subjects. Because of the nature of this survey, we used a signed consent form. After initial review, the Human Research Committee asked us to revise the consent form because they did not think it gave the volunteers sufficient information about the study. As you can see from the figure, we highlighted all of the specific areas about which the interviewer would ask questions in the consent form. The Human Research Committee approved this second version of the consent form.

Before beginning the interview, each interviewer read the consent form to the volunteer who then was free to ask any questions and to decide whether he or she would participate. If the volunteer did not wish to be part of the study, she or he declined to do so at this point and the interviewer left. If the volunteer agreed to become a respondent, she or he was given two copies of the consent form to sign. The respondent retained one copy and the other was brought back to us and filed separately from the respondent's interview. We did no cross-numbering or other linking of consent form and interview answer sheet. Thus respondents' identities were not indicated on their answer sheets, and their responses were indeed confidential. The whole purpose of this consent form was to ensure that the volunteer understood what the survey was about before she or he agreed to participate. No one was pressured to participate.

UNIVERSITY OF CALIFORNIA, SAN FRANCISCO

BERKELEY · DAVIS · IRVINE · LOS ANGELES · RIVERSIDE · SAN DIEGO · SAN FRANCISCO   SANTA BARBARA · SANTA CRUZ

SCHOOL OF NURSING
DEPARTMENT OF MENTAL HEALTH AND
COMMUNITY NURSING, ROOM N505-Y

SAN FRANCISCO, CALIFORNIA 94143

SENIOR RESOURCES SURVEY CONSENT FORM

THIS SURVEY IS BEING CONDUCTED FOR THE COUNTY AREA AGENCY ON
AGING BY STUDENTS FROM THE SCHOOL OF NURSING AT THE
UNIVERSITY OF CALIFORNIA IN SAN FRANCISCO.

THE SURVEY IS TO GATHER INFORMATION FROM OLDER ADULTS IN THE
COUNTY TO EVALUATE OUR KNOWLEDGE AND USE OF SOME OF THE
SERVICES AVAILABLE TO US. IT ALSO INCLUDES QUESTIONS ABOUT AGE,
INCOME LEVEL, MARITAL STATUS, LIVING ARRANGEMENTS, HEALTH,
SUPPORT SYSTEMS, INSURANCE, RETIREMENT, HOUSING, NEEDS, AND
PLANS IN CASE OF ILLNESS.

THE INTERVIEW WILL TAKE APPROXIMATELY FORTY-FIVE MINUTES. I MAY
STOP THE INTERVIEW AT ANY TIME AND I DO NOT HAVE TO ANSWER ANY
QUESTIONS I DON'T WANT TO. MY PARTICIPATION OR REFUSAL TO PARTI-
CIPATE WILL HAVE NO EFFECT ON MY ELIGIBILITY AT ANY TIME FOR ANY
SERVICES.

THE INTERVIEW WILL BE CONFIDENTIAL IN THAT I WILL NOT BE
IDENTIFIABLE IN ANY WAY IN ANY REPORT OF THIS SURVEY.

IF I HAVE ANY QUESTIONS ABOUT THE INTERVIEW I MAY CALL EITHER
SARAH ARCHER AT (Phone number) OR ELLEN CAULFIELD AT
(Phone number).

HAVING BEEN TOLD ALL OF THE ABOVE, I CONSENT TO BE INTERVIEWED.

            Date   Signature

Because we knew who the respondents in the assessment were, considerable precautions had to be taken to assure confidentiality. As noted, there was no cross-coding between signed consent forms and completed answer sheets. Answer sheets were code numbered to identify the area of the county in which the respondent lived so that we could compare data from the northern, middle, and southern areas. Identification cards with name, address, and directions to the place of interview were kept separate from answer sheets, and the cards were destroyed immediately after the assessment was completed. Signed consent forms were filed in Sarah Archer's office, separate from everything else.

We were concerned that some of the respondents might have questions about the assessment or the questions they had been asked after the interviewer had left. For this reason the consent form contained the names and phone numbers of both Sarah Archer and Ellen Caulfield, the AAA executive, in case respondents wished to call either one. As far as we know, no one called with questions.

Administration of the instrument

As noted, the media announcements of the assessment invited interested seniors to call their local information and referral service and leave their name and address. People at the referral services were instructed on what information to record (box, below). When this proved to provide too few potential participants, other agencies in the county were contacted and asked for referrals of people who were known to dining sites, blood pressure clinics, and congregate housing sites whom we could contact to invite to participate. Although our proportion of successfully completed interviews was higher from persons who called in to volunteer than from those whose names were given to us by other agencies, not all of the volunteers were interviewed.

INSTRUCTIONS FOR RECORDING INTAKE CALLS

When a call comes in from an individual who would like to participate in the AAA Senior Resources Survey, please do the following:

1. On the 5 × 8 cards take:
   Name
   Address
   City, Zip code
   Telephone number
   Referral source
2. Inform the individual that someone will return the call early in April
3. Thank them for calling

Thank you for helping!

There were several reasons for this. There was a time lag between the volunteer's call and student's contact to arrange an interview. In the meantime, some of the volunteers had forgotten about the assessment or were no longer available for interview. Other declined to participate when the assessment was further explained to them. A few declined to be interviewed because their health status had changed and they were "not up to it." Contact with persons referred to us by agencies was more problematic since we were initiating contact with them. A good deal more salespersonship was needed to interest these persons in participating than was the case for those who volunteered. Reference to a familiar agency does not always guarantee cooperation.

We gave the students the names of the people who had volunteered or had been referred. Their first job was to contact the person, to explain the evaluation, and to arrange a mutually convenient time and place for the interview. The class schedule allowed one afternoon a week for the interviewing (a 4-hour period). If arrangements were made between the student and volunteer at other times, that was up to them. As sometimes happens in the community, plans were made and the student went out to the home to find no one there. On the whole, however, most appointments were kept.

Once in the home, assuring privacy for the interview had to be considered. The potentially sensitive nature of some of the interview questions prompted us to instruct the interviewers to find a place where they could talk alone to respondents so that the respondents' answers were not influenced by the presence or comments of other people. In circumstances in which the person lived alone and had no visitors at the time that the interview was scheduled to take place, privacy assurance was not an issue. In circumstances where the person lived with family members or other people or who had attendant care, the interviewer requested a place where the respondent and interviewer could talk alone. Curiosity being what it is, a few persons volunteered to be interviewed after their spouses had been.

The interviewer read the consent form to the senior and answered any questions. Once the two consent forms were signed, the interview could begin. Interviewers stressed the necessity of sticking to the questions as they were asked. They were instructed to advise respondents: "if some of the questions on the interview make you think of other areas, we can talk about them after the interview is over." Many of the interviewers found that respondents did indeed want to talk about other areas. Thus the time that the interviewers spent with respondents varied from 35 to 90 minutes.

The interviewer then conducted the interview, reading the questions exactly as they appeared. Respondents were given information on cards so that they could read the choices of possible answers. Standard definitions of services and specific probing questions were written out for the interviewers to ensure reliability. Once the formal interview was completed, the interviewer was free to talk with the respondent about anything he or she wished. As you can see from the questionnaire on pp. 194-205 there are many questions that could cause respondents to think of other topics they would want to talk about. Also, the elderly, particularly those who live alone, are often lonely and welcome opportunities to talk. Respondents knew their interviewers were nurses and so might have been more inclined to discuss health concerns with them.

Anticipating this, we emphasized to the students that they were there in the capacity of interviewers, not as nurses. They were responsible for referring any problems to community agencies or to discuss problems they learned about with the graduate student supervisors, but they themselves were not to function in the role of the nurse. We provided them with a copy of services in the community for the seniors and also with emergency numbers. There were a few referrals but, fortunately, no crisis.

Access and entry

In the few years between the needs and life-style assessment and this study, NDC had expanded its programs in the county to three adult day-care centers and an in-home services project. Sarah Archer was on NDC's board and was a vice-chair of the AAA's Commission on Aging. Carole Kelly had spent her master's program residencies with NDC at the day-care centers and, by the time the surveys were being done, had also become a member of the Commission on Aging. We had built a foundation over a period of time and had been very careful to protect our credibility in the community.

The fact that nurses were the interviewers also contributed to the credibility of the survey. There is a trusting relationship between the public and the nursing profession particularly in the public or community health field. Nurses appear free of vested interest and have the advantage of not being seen as a group that can jeopardize an individual's income status. Social workers tend to be seen more skeptically because of their connections with eligibility workers and with Medicaid. Nurses are also healers and counselors.

After we realized that there were not going to be enough volunteers from the community at large, we decided to go to the community agencies (see Fig. 3, p. 34). The advantage of knowing personnel in most of these agencies firsthand did not entirely free us from the gatekeeper's syndrome. In fact, it was made clear to us that as insiders we should understand their concerns and we did. Seniors are constantly complaining of the "studying us" syndrome.[3] We appreciated that problem. We also knew that little quality study of the seniors' needs had been done on a community basis and that future planning and program development was dependent on some sound source of information. The fact that we were able to deal with the gatekeepers on a one-to-one basis helped us immensely to gain access, particularly in cases in which we had to seek referrals of potential participants. For example, after the

UNIVERSITY OF CALIFORNIA, SAN FRANCISCO

BERKELEY · DAVIS · IRVINE · LOS ANGELES · RIVERSIDE · SAN DIEGO · SAN FRANCISCO   SANTA BARBARA · SANTA CRUZ

SAN FRANCISCO, CALIFORNIA 94143

SCHOOL OF NURSING
DEPARTMENT OF MENTAL HEALTH AND
COMMUNITY NURSING, ROOM N505-Y

February 23, 1981

Dear Colleagues:

The County Area Agency on Aging is working with the School of Nursing,
University of California, San Francisco, in developing a survey to evaluate
older adults' knowledge and utilization of the county's senior services.
The details of the project are contained in the enclosed announcement.

We need your assistance in getting information about the survey out
to the community. Thus we request that you alert staff, volunteers, and
clients about the survey. Please share the announcement with these groups
and encourage them to inform seniors who might be willing to volunteer to
participate.

If you have a bulletin or newsletter that will go out between now and
the middle of April, please include this announcement and the instructions
for contacting Information and Referral.

The survey will also serve as an educational and outreach service for
the agencies providing services for the elderly since a copy of SOS will be
left with every volunteer respondent. The results of the survey should be
available from the Area Agency on Aging in the Fall.

Thank you for your assistance in this project.

Sincerely,

Sarah E. Archer, R.N., Dr.P.H.
Associate Professor and Vice-Chair,
    County Commission on Aging and Chair,
Health Committee

SEA/md

interviews began and contact was to be made with some of the meal sites, some of the graduate students went out to the meal sites and talked with the site coordinators and the participants. This personal touch was appreciated and contributed to more seniors volunteering to participate in the survey.

Because some of the agencies from which we sought volunteers were also agencies being evaluated in the study, the staff of these agencies viewed us as a threat (see Chapter 5). We did our best to reassure them and to discuss the process carefully with them. Again, we cannot emphasize too much the importance of the regard given to members of colleague agencies who can so effectively limit or facilitate access to potential subjects for community assessments. A copy of the letter we sent to colleagues in community agencies to introduce the survey to them and to request their help can be seen on p. 181.

ANALYSIS OF DATA

Since the answer sheets that the interviewers completed were carefully pre-coded, the transfer of data to the computer was relatively easy. Again we used the Statistical Package in the Social Sciences,[4] since it was appropriate for the kinds of analyses we wanted to do. Graduate students began the data analysis process under Sally Bisch's guidance. One of our objectives was for the master's students to gain at least beginning familiarity with computer use as part of their experience. Although they did have some opportunity to begin the analysis, computer complications and the end of the academic quarter terminated their involvement. Before the course ended, the graduate students were able to present initial frequencies and a few crosstabulations to the entire class. This provided all of the students with some feeling that they had seen much of the project from beginning to end.

With the help of one of the master's students, Meladee Stankus, whose husband is a programmer, we completed the final analysis of the data and wrote the report during the summer of 1981. The reality is that, although there were many times when we wished we had more help in that process, we were much aware of the disadvantages of having too many workers. One example of this is that some of the computer runs had been corrected differently than had others, since a number of people had been involved. Once we caught these differences, we were able to correct them and make a comparable analysis. Even though there were only 138 usable respondents in the study, they provided us with a mountain of data. Although we completed the report for the AAA in terms of what they wanted, there are opportunities for secondary analysis of these data, just as there were from the first assessment.

USES OF THE EVALUATION FINDINGS

Carole Kelly presented the final report to the Commission on Aging in October 1981 (see pp. 206-239). The AAA used the data in developing the 1982-83 Area Plan, which was their objective in asking that the evaluation be conducted. The

AAA's planner, Lynn Friss, prepared an executive summary for distribution. Carole Kelly used this material in her presentations of the assessment to a number of agencies.

The data from this evaluation were compared with those generated in the one done in the rural western part of the community. Many interesting similarities and differences were found between the urban and rural areas. These findings have been helpful in developing appropriate services for the elderly in both communities.

The recommendations generated by the assessment's findings were referred to the Commission on Aging's Planning Committee, which used them for considering specific kinds of needs and the programs or other approaches that might best address them. As is almost always the case, as the commission worked with the results of both our evaluation and the one from the rural area, they became aware of the need for additional information to aid them in planning. If only time and money were available.

THE PROCESS IN RETROSPECT

The evaluation met the objectives of the AAA for providing it with current material to use for its area plan. As an educational experience for the undergraduate students, it was far less successful than we had hoped. Part of the problems were created by the sheer number of undergraduate students (39) and the fact that virtually none of them had had any kind of extrainstitutional experience, although they all were registered nurses. The access problems we encountered created a great deal of confusion and frustration for everyone. The constraint of having to finish all of the interviewing and as much of the data analysis as possible before the end of the spring quarter placed a real stress on us all. In that respect our planning of the timing of the assessment was faulty. We should have allowed at least two quarters and preferably three for such an undertaking. However, such a time frame would not fit into the undergraduate's carefully constructed curriculum. If only our foresight could be as clear as our hindsight!

•   •   •

Collaborating with members of community systems to bring about change, as with most process, is best learned by doing. No matter how many of them one does, each brings new rewards, challenges, and problems. They are never dull. Our intent in including these two examples of actual evaluations is to ground many of the principles and processes presented elsewhere in this book in reality. Now read our example and go try one yourselves!

INTERVIEWER PREPARATION

Ruth Fleshman prepared and conducted the 6 hour interviewer preparation. The following is the format that she used. You may wish to use all or part of it.

PROCEDURES FOR INTERVIEWERS

Ruth P. Fleshman, RN, PhD

Persons to be interviewed

You will be given the name, address, zip code, and phone number of older persons who have agreed to be interviewed. Phone them to make an appointment for your visit. Introduce yourself by name and identify yourself as the nursing student carrying out the older adults' survey for the county Area Agency on Aging and the University of California at San Francisco. Arrange for a mutually agreeable time for the interview, which should take no more than 45 minutes. Obtain directions for getting to the respondent's home. KEEP THE APPOINTMENT AS ARRANGED. If you cannot humanly do so, phone the respondent as soon as you realize you are not going to be able to arrive as scheduled and make a new appointment.

Initiating the interview

On arriving, introduce yourself by name and explain that you are the nursing student from the University of California participating in the survey of older adults for the county Area Agency on Aging. Confirm that the person you are talking to is the person whose name you got to be a respondent.

> Hello, Mrs. Jones? [Yes] I'm Ann Smith, the nursing student from the University of California who called you last week. I'm here to carry out the survey on service agencies that's being done for the Area Agency on Aging.

It is important for both of you to be comfortable during the interview. Most subjects are likely to suggest sitting in the living room. But be adaptable to wherever the person wishes to be. Be sure you are in a chair that allows you to write on the answer sheet, be close enough to the respondent to hand over the various response cards, and to hear each other easily. Be aware that older people may have a hearing deficit they don't acknowledge, so be prepared to adapt your volume level so the respondent can hear you well.

Be sure you and the interviewee are alone during the interview. The person's spouse or caretaker may want to remain to help. However, there is sometimes a problem of such people wanting to answer *for* the person. Since this survey is to get the interviewee's answers, you should thank them for the offer but say it is more important to get the exact thought of the person being interviewed. (Another reason you should not mention is that the answers to some of the questions might well be changed if there is another significant person within hearing.) One successful tactic may be to specify that the interview will last 45 minutes and so the other person can feel free to go out or otherwise occupy his or her time knowing you will be there that long. If that doesn't work, offer to interview that other person after completing this one.

Conducting a research interview

Nurses interview people all the time within our professional activities. Even there, we have several different purposes in doing so. In some cases, we want to get basic objective facts to fill out a form, for example, or the identifying material for a fact sheet or health history. At other times we want to get at how people feel about certain things, either very particular events or, with a more psychological orientation, how they respond and feel about things in general. And some interviews are conducted as a therapeutic means of allowing individuals to ventilate. In almost every instance, we are constantly alert for indications that our professional service is needed; we are constantly ready to gear up our nursing interventions.

Unlike a nursing interview, this research interview is *not* the basis for any nursing intervention. It is designated to get objective data, brief responses to a standard set of questions. These responses must be capable of being categorized in a limited number and counted in order to give us a picture of how our subjects as a group responded. For that reason the questionnaire is set up to have answers recorded by a numerical code. That means we cannot use all the detailed anecdotes that a lot of people want to tell us. (That's a different kind of interview than this one.) If you find yourself talking with a "rambler," you may want to say something like "I don't want to take up too much time, so I'd like to go on with the next question."

You may well find yourself in a situation that suggests the need for varying degrees of assistance, and it will be very hard to keep from wanting to fall back into your nurse role. It is crucial that you avoid doing so. It is also very hard not to want to. Please try to hold on to your clinical impulse until the end of the form. At that point, there is a question about the person's most pressing need. If that or any other problem has become painfully clear, you can point out an appropriate service in the community resource pamphlet, which you can *then* give the person. Because you are *not* in that person's home as a nurse, you do not have either the right or the obligation to intervene. However, if you are seriously upset by something you have observed, please discuss it with your graduate student supervisor who is scheduled to be available to you during your interview time. Keep her phone number with you in case you need to call her either right then or after leaving the interview.

If you feel that something in the interview situation has caused a problem of serious nature for the respondent, either try to make amends or break off the questioning. Occasionally older people, especially those who have had strokes, may begin to cry for no apparent reason or for some cause apparently so trivial that it seems illogical. Try not to appear upset yourself, reassure the person, pause briefly, then if calm does not return, ask if he/she wants to discontinue or will be able to go on in a while.

It is possible that some respondents will get angry about being interviewed. A certain number of people have become hostile to the idea of research or may be manifesting some of the anti-government spirit that is rife right now. To the extent possible, try to avoid arguing. Instead try to explain, as feasible, that this project is being done with volunteers so there is no special taxpayer money going for research. Nor is this a purely academic exercise; the purpose of the survey is to provide a sensible basis for planning health services for county older adults.

Be sure to give no sense that there is a right or wrong answer. It is important to get each person to feel that whatever answer is given is important (and it is). By making encouraging noises, like "Um humm" or "Yes," you give evidence that you are paying attention. In those cases when the answer is completely off the track from the question, you may, without suggesting they are wrong, get them back by saying something like "I guess I didn't ask that one right; what I meant was . . ." and then reask the question, emphasizing the salient word, using one of the given probes, or even reading the list of answers from which you expect them to pick. (That last choice is not one to be used very often, but may need to be used from sheer desperation.)

Explaining the interview

The ethics of research requires that subjects understand the purpose of the interview. That explanation has been approved by a committee specially designated by the University. It is necessary both to give the subject that explanation in written form and to read it aloud before asking that the subject sign the form giving consent to be interviewed. (Some older people get very wary about legal-sounding terms, especially when they are then required to sign something. After reading the consent form (see p. 177), you may find it necessary to reexplain its content in less imposing language. Some subjects will still refuse to sign the consent form even though agreeing to be interviewed. This is a dilemma and if it occurs very often, we will have to discuss the problem with the Research Committee. In the meantime, try to persuade them to sign but do not use unethical means to do so. There can be no hint of disapproval or of any consequenees to the subject for such lack of cooperation.)

After signing, each subject is allowed to keep a copy of the written explanation to look over at any later time and to keep in mind what it was they agreed to do. Note the provision there for phone numbers they can call for any additional information they might wish.

You will note that part of the explanation is that all responses remain confidential and will not be individually identifiable in the final report. The mechanism we use to guarantee that is to assign each interviewee a code number to be written onto the answer sheet so names are never used after the interview is finished. No record is kept of numbers assigned to individuals and no name should be placed on the answer sheet.

You are obligated to maintain that confidentiality. You must not share with the interview subject what any other interviewee has said; that would be a clear indicator that you are not maintaining someone else's privacy. But you also must not share this information with anyone outside the project. Like any professional, you have the right to information that people consider "personal" *only* if you keep that information from becoming known in ways that could have consequences for the interviewee or his/her significant others. (We have a tendency to "talk shop" among ourselves, using identifying names. And when this is overheard in the halls or elevators, it does much to destroy the belief that health professionals can be trusted to keep private matters private. Please try not to destroy what little credibility researchers have left.)

Besides explaining the overall purpose of the interview, you may also be asked to explain some particular question. Each is specifically discussed in the section on the survey questions (see pp. 188-191). In general, items are of three kinds. The first are aimed at what the person knows about the service resources in the county. That of course is the main focus of the survey. A number of questions get at demographic information about the person: age, race, sex, income, etc. These questions are intended to give perspective on the characteristics of the people answering our questions. This way we can compare groups of older people within our sample as well as compare them to the general population of older adults in the county. (Some people get nervous about questions of income.) For that reason the only specific money question (14) asks only if he/she is above the official poverty line. In addition, there are some questions that ask for subjective answers, preferences for instance about living arrangements, retirement, and health. These are the kinds of items that will be useful in planning services for what people say they want.

Asking the questions

The goal of our survey is to collect as many responses as possible to a standardized series of questions about what older county residents know and how they use a range of health and human services in the county. The questions on the survey have been written to be as clearly understandable by any average person as possible. They have been tried out and found to give the kinds of answers we can manage with the computer. Thus it is very important to ask the questions exactly as written each time you interview someone. If the questions were reworded from one subject to another, it would not be possible to guarantee that the answers collected could be compared. Similarly, you need to ask the questions in the same order each time. They have been placed in the order given so that each subject's reaction to one question will similarly flavor the response to the next one. If you move them about, we can't be sure that any given response has had the same emotional tone from one subject to another.

On the interview form, you will note that the material you are to ask the subject is written in normal typed form. The instructions to the interviewer ARE TYPED IN CAPITAL LETTERS; these are not to be read aloud. In addition, after certain questions, there are added words saying SUGGESTED STANDARD PROBE. These are phrases tested out to help the interviewee better understand what it is we are asking for. If the subject answers freely, don't bother using the probe. If, however, they seem not to understand or are answering with material that doesn't fit the answers, the probe should be used to get them back on track.

Recording answers

Be prepared to write down answers as soon as you ask the questions. Have your writing implement ready to go. However, it is important to not be too businesslike: look up at your interviewee and keep an interested expression on your face, a slight smile perhaps, to encourage a response. Eye contact also encourages the person to feel confident about answering.

Mark the code number in the appropriate box on the answer sheet as soon as the person answers. Do not ask the next question until you have recorded the answer to the previous one. You may think you can keep several answers in mind, but it's just too easy to get confused or distracted.

Any coded questionnaire can present only a limited number of choices for answers. Thus you may be required to force code a response into that category that most closely resembles the answer you are hearing. In some cases, there will not be an acceptably close one given. In the questions that ask for more or less open responses, there is always one reply at the end that is "Other (SPECIFY)". When this is used, try to select one or two words that characterize the answer you are hearing and, after marking the answer box with the code number that matches that response, write the question number down in the lower left hand open area of the answer sheet and follow it with the words you believe reflects the answer. (You may need to use the reverse of the answer sheet if you get a lot of "Other (SPECIFY)" replies.) We often find that eventually another category of answer begins to emerge from such responses and this is one of the things that makes research interesting.

Cards

Each of you will have three 5- by 8-inch cards to use with your interviews. These are for questions 1, 2, and 14 (see pp. 195, 196, and 199). They contain lists the respondent will answer questions about and serve to help the person focus on what is being asked. New information is not always clearly understood when it is presented in only one way—and that can be either only in print or only in spoken form. Double forms of presentation increase the likelihood of understanding. This is particularly important when the questioning is as complicated as in 1 and 2. Of course, the person has to be able to read the lettering. Unless the person is announced to be blind, you will need to test this. Hand the person the first card and follow the process laid out in the questionnaire instrument (p. 194). Note the process, marked with 3 asterisks, to be used with a respondent who cannot read.

Survey questions

Keeping in mind the overall goal of this survey (pp. 170-171), let us now review the specific questions and any special points about recording responses to them.

Question 1. This presents a range of community services available in the county (see box, p. 189). At the top of each column are questions that need to be asked about each of the services. The first, "Are you aware of this," if answered *no*, would mean

SERVICES FOR THE ELDERLY

1. **Information and referral:** a telephone referral service that provides information about services for the elderly
2. **Legal assistance:** a service that provides legal assistance to the elderly
3. **Transportation:** bus services to meal sites and programs as well as to some appointments
4. **Day care for the elderly:** supervised day program for the frail elderly that provides health counseling, programs, as well as respite for the family
5. **Meal sites:** federally funded noon meal program; also a dinner program at one site
6. **In-home meals:** home-delivered meals for shut-ins
7. **Senior employment:** employment, referral, and counseling services for older adults
8. **Recreation programs:** senior clubs and organizations that offer recreational programs for those 55 and over
9. **Public health nurse:** a nurse from the county health department who provides direct and indirect health care, education, and screening for county residents
10. **Senior health project:** health assessment program held at various locations in the community, providing counseling and group health education as well as referral service
11. **Blood pressure clinic:** blood pressure checks, well-person counseling, and nutritional counseling program done on an appointment basis
12. **Health counseling:** counseling services available for the elderly from a variety of sources, e.g., public health nurse, Nursing Dynamics, health educator
13. **Exercise classes:** classes available at a variety of locations that are designed for the older adult
14. **In-home services:** a service that offers to link clients to in-home care providers
15. **Friendly visitor:** a program that is available to the elderly in the county that provides a companion to visit an individual in the home to try to alleviate loneliness
16. **Adult protective services:** a service provided by the county health department that is available for the protection of adults from abuse
17. **Supportive services from churches:** services that range from home visits to transportation and meal preparation to counseling
18. **Outreach:** the program that attempts to let the older adults in the community know that there are services available to them
19. **Nursing home omsbudsman:** a program that provides protection and support to individuals in nursing homes by advocating for quality services in the institutions

that the other questions about it are not answerable. Please note that the first, second, fourth, and fifth columns take only a *yes* (1) or *no* (2) response. The third and sixth ask for another kind of answer; the coded list at the top has several answers from which to choose. If the gist of the response matches one of those given, enter its number into the appropriate box on the answer sheet. If the response does not match the choices, mark the box 8 and enter in the blank area a word or brief phrase that most closely characterizes the answer. (Be sure to put down the question number with the answer.)

Be alert to possibilities that your respondent is unclear about the differences

---

COMMUNITY MENTAL HEALTH

1. **Crisis unit:** a 24-hour short-term facility at the county general hospital for psychiatric emergencies
2. **Outpatient units:** outpatient clinics providing psychiatric care
3. **Transitional services:** after-care for patients who have recently been discharged from psychiatric facilities
4. **Companion program:** a program within transitional services that matches clients with volunteers who provide support while clients are coping with their return to the community
5. **Developmental disabilities:** a program that provides case management to families and clients with developmental disabilities
6. **Mobile geriatric evaluation team:** a home-visit program for the elderly in which a nurse assesses problems and advises action without making a psychiatric diagnosis
7. **Home visits for older adults:** a program in which some therapists and crisis unit outreach workers make home visits

---

between 9, 10, 11, and 12. There are commonalities there, and you may need to ask where these services were found. (PHNs take blood pressures in their own practices; PHNs work for the Senior Health Project and take blood pressures; blood pressures are taken in various locales such as the Heart Association, the health counseling program at the senior center, and even in some fire houses.) The same goes for 17 and 18, since churches do outreach.

Question 2. The same questions are to be asked about the various elements of the Community Mental Health Department (see box, above).

Questions 3 through 6. Questions 3 through 6 are basic demographic identifiers. Enter the code number that reflects the age given by your respondent, the sex, marital status, and race. (Note the possibility of some other ethnic identity; if this is used, mark 7 in the box and write the response in the lower-lefthand blank space. Be sure to number it Q.6.

Questions 7 through 11. Questions 7 through 11 ask about housing and living arrangements. This is a major problem area for the elderly and we need basic information about how our respondents are housed. Notice that if the person answers *no* to question 8, you are instructed to skip to question 10; if *yes* to question 9, to skip to question 12. This pattern of alternative questions will recur, so watch out for it.

Questions 12 and 13. Questions 12 and 13 ask if there are arrangments that would be preferred. These are examples of why the respondent should be alone with you since there would be less likelihood of a yes if not.

Questions 14 through 16. Questions 14 through 16 ask about sources of income and whether the monthly total is above the official poverty level. Each type of income source has its own yes/no answer, so please enter either *1* or *2* in each of the boxes for question 14.

Question 17. Question 17 asks the length of local residence to establish how respondent compares with other aged in the county.

Questions 18 through 24. Questions 18 through 22 ask facts about employment status and, for those who are retired, asks about the negative aspects of having had to retire. Questions 23 and 24 seek to learn attitudes of those still employed to their work situation.

Question 25. Question 25 is intended to gauge how a person evaluates his/her own health. Notice that the key word here is *health;* some respondents tend to get off on other aspects of their circumstances, especially in relation to finances. If you feel this is happening, emphasize that you are asking only about their health in relation to others their own age.

Questions 26 and 27. Questions 26 and 27 ask about extent of health insurance coverage. Each type has its own yes/no answer, so please enter either *1* or *2* in each of the boxes for question 26. Note that 26-e refers only to private insurance; mark this answer if they give the name of a firm that carries some health policy such as Mutual of Indiana, Metropolitan, etc.

Question 28. Question 28 asks about interval since seeing a physician.

Questions 29 and 30. Questions 29 and 30 ask the person to speculate about care arrangements in case of dependency and how this would be managed if home were the preferred arrangement.

Question 31. Question 31 asks if the person would want to continue living in a state of total dependence.

Questions 32 through 35. Question 32 asks about the availability of a confidant, and questions 33 and 34 ask the relationship and its supportiveness. If not supportive enough, question 35 asks for possible reasons. The answer may be several of those given or one not already listed. Please answer each area *yes* or *no.* If the answer is number 35-i, write any additional type of reason that doesn't approximate those given in the lower left corner.

Question 36. Question 36 asks the respondent to identify one problem (ONLY ONE). After getting a response, please give them a copy of the community resource pamphlet. Explain that this is a fairly old version but the newer one is still being held up for lack of funding, so they should check out the currency of any number they want to contact. Please write the actual word user *under* the box with the coded answer.

Answer sheet

At the top of the sheet there are six code items to be filled out before returning each form. These include the ID number assigned to this sheet by your graduate student supervisor and the last three digits of your respondent's zip code. The other four items come from answers given in the course of the interview; the number of the item is in parentheses. (These aid computer card punching.) Please note there is no place for the respondent's name; this is to protect confidentiality.

Coding space for answers for each of the 19 services for the elderly is provided under question 1. Coding space for answers for the 7 community mental health services is found under question 2. Notice that items 13 and 36 have a divided space; the coded responses to these questions require two digits.

Blank areas are left on the lower left corner and the narrow space under item 36. These and the back of the sheet are available for recording whatever answers respondents give that fail to approximate the precoded categories of answers that have been given. Be sure to mark the item box with the appropriate number for "Other (SPECIFY)" and on the back enter the question number and the briefest summary of the actual answer given to that item.

Every box on the answer sheet must have some number in it to be complete. When you have finished your interviews, look over the sheet to see if you have failed to ask a question. Fill in all the numbers at that time so you will have no reason to have to call back.

ANSWER SHEET

Subject ID #_____   ZIP code (last 3 digits only)_____
(3) Age category _____   (5) Marital status _____
(4) Sex _____   (15) Income Level _____

Question 1

	Aware	Used	Why not	Other	Would you	Why not
1.						
2.						
3.						
4.						
5.						
6.						
7.						
8.						
9.						
10.						
11.						
12.						
13.						
14.						
15.						
16.						
17.						
18.						
19.						

Question 2

	Aware	Used	Why not	Other	Would you	Why not
1.						
2.						
3.						
4.						
5.						
6.						
7.						

Questions 3-36

3.	22.	34.
4.	23.	35a.
5.	24.	b.
6.	25.	c.
7.	26a.	d.
8.	b.	e.
9.	c.	f.
10.	d.	g.
11.	e.	h.
12.	f.	i.
13.	g.	36.
14a.	h.	
b.	27.	
c.	28.	
d.	29.	
e.	30a.	
f.	b.	
g.	c.	
h.	d.	
i.	e.	
15.	f.	
16.	31.	
17.	32.	
18.	33a.	
19.	b.	
20.	c.	
21a.	d.	
b.	e.	
c.	f.	
d.	g.	
e.	h.	
f.	i.	

Ending the interview

After giving the respondent the community resource pamphlet and doing whatever seems indicated to help them use it as effectively as possible (see p. 191 under Question 36 for warning on possible obsolescence), thank the respondent pleasantly and ask if there are any questions that might be answered. Deal with them if you can; those that you cannot answer should be referred to the appropriate answerer and tell the respondent you will have that person respond to the question. Pass the question along to your graduate student supervisor with the phone number of the person asking it. Do not include the interview code number with that information.

If there are no questions or loose ends, thank the respondent and leave.

THE SURVEY INSTRUMENT

INTERVIEWER INSTRUCTION: HAND CARD 1 TO RESPONDENT,*** THEN READ THE FOLLOWING:

We realize some older adults have difficulty with their eyesight.

Are you able to read this card?

CHECK ONE   YES 1

NO 2

NO RESPONSE 9

IF YES, PROCEED.

IF NO, WHEN CARD IS TO BE USED FOLLOW SPECIAL INSTRUCTIONS.***

TO EACH RESPONDENT SAY:

1. There are many services available for older adults in this county. We would like to see if you are familiar with these services or have used them. We are also interested in knowing why you have not used them.

TO EACH RESPONDENT SAY: Please look at the list of services I have given you. We will go over these one by one.

***SPECIAL INSTRUCTION:

TO THIS RESPONDENT SAY: I will go over a list of services slowly once. Then I will go over these services *again* and ask you about each one.

INTERVIEWER CODE:

MARK APPROPRIATE NUMBER

Yes 1   Have private resources 6

No 2   No transportation 7

Not interested 3   Other (SPECIFY) 8

Not needed 4   No response (N/R) 9

Too ill 5

OTHER, MARK APPROPRIATE NUMBER AND SPECIFY REASON ON CODE SHEET.

CARD 1. SERVICES FOR ELDERLY

1. INFORMATION AND REFERRAL
2. LEGAL ASSISTANCE
3. TRANSPORTATION
4. DAY CARE FOR THE ELDERLY
5. MEAL SITES
6. IN-HOME MEALS
7. SENIOR EMPLOYMENT
8. RECREATION PROGRAMS
9. PUBLIC HEALTH NURSE
10. SENIOR HEALTH PROJECT
11. BLOOD PRESSURE CLINIC
12. HEALTH COUNSELING
13. EXERCISE CLASSES
14. IN-HOME SERVICES
15. FRIENDLY VISITORS
16. ADULT PROTECTIVE SERVICES
17. SUPPORT SERVICES FROM CHURCH GROUPS
18. OUTREACH
19. NURSING HOME OMBUDSMAN

Service	Are you aware of this?	Have you used it?	If no, why not?	Do you know others who have used it?	Would you use it if needed?	If no, why not?
Information and referral	——	——	——	——	——	——
Legal assistance	——	——	——	——	——	——
Transportation	——	——	——	——	——	——
Day care for the elderly	——	——	——	——	——	——
Meal sites	——	——	——	——	——	——
In-home meals	——	——	——	——	——	——
Senior employment	——	——	——	——	——	——
Recreation programs	——	——	——	——	——	——
Public health nurse	——	——	——	——	——	——
Senior health project	——	——	——	——	——	——
Blood pressure clinic	——	——	——	——	——	——
Health counseling	——	——	——	——	——	——
Exercise classes	——	——	——	——	——	——
In-home services	——	——	——	——	——	——
Friendly visitors	——	——	——	——	——	——
Adult protective services	——	——	——	——	——	——
Support services from church groups	——	——	——	——	——	——
Outreach	——	——	——	——	——	——
Nursing home ombudsman	——	——	——	——	——	——

CARD 2. COMMUNITY MENTAL HEALTH SERVICES

1. CRISIS UNIT
2. OUTPATIENT UNITS
3. TRANSITIONAL SERVICES
4. THE COMPANION PROGRAM
5. DEVELOPMENTAL DISABILITIES UNIT
6. MOBILE GERIATRIC EVALUATION TEAM
7. HOME VISITS FOR OLDER ADULTS

Service	Are you aware of this?	Have you used it?	If no, why not?	Do you know others who have used it?	Would you use it if needed?	If no, why not?
Crisis unit	_____	_____	_____	_____	_____	_____
Outpatient units	_____	_____	_____	_____	_____	_____
Transitional services	_____	_____	_____	_____	_____	_____
The companion program	_____	_____	_____	_____	_____	_____
Developmental disabilities unit	_____	_____	_____	_____	_____	_____
Mobile geriatric evaluation team	_____	_____	_____	_____	_____	_____
Home visits for older adults	_____	_____	_____	_____	_____	_____

INTERVIEWER INSTRUCTION: HAND CARD 2 TO RESPONDENT***

TO EACH RESPONDENT SAY:

2. There are special programs designed for older adults by Community Mental Health Services. Would you look at this list and see if you are familiar with them?

***SPECIAL INSTRUCTION:

TO THIS RESPONDENT SAY: I will go over a list of services designed by Community Mental Health Services for older adults slowly first. Then I will go over them once more and ask you about your familiarity with each.

INTERVIEWER CODE: CONTINUE AS IN QUESTION 1.

TO EACH RESPONDENT SAY: This part of the questionnaire deals with some background information we need from you to find out something about the people over 60 in this county.

INTERVIEWER TO CIRCLE RIGHT NUMBER

3. How old are you?
   INTERVIEWER: GIVE AGE RANGE

60-64	1
65-74	2
75-84	3
85-100	4
N/R	9

4. RESPONDENT'S SEX—
   INTERVIEWER: CIRCLE UNLESS UNSURE—THEN ASK

Male	1
Female	2
N/R	9

5. INTERVIEWER: What is your marital status?
   IF ANSWER IS "SINGLE," ASK RESPONDENT TO BE SPECIFIC

Never married	1
Separated	2
Divorced	3
Widowed	4
Married, living with spouse	5
Married, spouse in hospital or nursing home	6
N/R	9

6. Which of the following identifies you?

White	1
Black	2
Hispanic/Latino	3
Chinese	4
Japanese	5
Native American (Indian)	6
Other (SPECIFY)	7
N/R	9

7. With whom do you live?

Alone	1
Husband	2
Wife	3
Son	4
Daughter	5
Friend	6
Other relative	7
Other (SPECIFY)	8
N/R	9

8. Do you own your own home?

Yes 1
No 2
N/R 9
(IF NO, SKIP TO QUESTION 10)

IF YES, ASK:
9. Is it paid for?

Yes 1
No 2
N/R 9
(IF YES, SKIP TO QUESTION 12)

10. Do you rent?

Yes 1
No 2
N/R 9
(IF YES, SKIP TO QUESTION 12)

IF NO, ASK:
11. If you don't own or rent, what living arrangements do you have?

Living with relative 1
Pay room and board 2
Share a house 3
Caretaker in exchange for place to live . . . 4
Other (SPECIFY) 5
N/R 9

12. Would you prefer different living arrangements?

Yes 1
No 2
N/R 9
(IF NO, SKIP TO QUESTION 14)

IF YES, ASK:
13. What would your ideal housing accommodations be?
    (SUGGESTED STANDARD PROBE: For example, would you rather be living
    in any of the following:)

Apartment 01
Single room 02
Retirement center 03
Board and care 04
Share housing 05
Room in family's home 06
Own home 07
Nursing home 08
Hotel 09
Condominium 10
Other (SPECIFY) 11
N/R 99

```
┌──────────────────────────────────────────────────────────────────────┐
│                                                                        │
│                      CARD 3. INCOME SOURCES                            │
│                                                                        │
│   EMPLOYMENT                                                           │
│   SOCIAL SECURITY                                                      │
│   GOVERNMENT PENSION                                                   │
│   OLD AGE ASSISTANCE (SSI)                                             │
│   PRIVATE PENSION                                                      │
│   INTEREST, INVESTMENT, OR RENTALS                                     │
│   RELATIVES                                                            │
│   SAVINGS WITHDRAWALS, SALE OF REAL ESTATE, OR                         │
│       CASHING BONDS                                                    │
│   OTHER                                                                │
│                                                                        │
└──────────────────────────────────────────────────────────────────────┘
```

INTERVIEWER INSTRUCTION: HAND CARD 3 TO RESPONDENT***
14. From which of the following sources do you get your monthly income?
    CIRCLE *ALL* ANSWERS GIVEN

***SPECIAL INSTRUCTION:

TO THIS RESPONDENT SAY: I will go over a list of income sources. Please tell me
    which of the following contribute to your monthly income?

Employment	Yes	1
	No	2
Social security	Yes	1
	No	2
Government pension	Yes	1
	No	2
Old age assistance (SSI)	Yes	1
	No	2
Private pension	Yes	1
	No	2
Interest, investments, or rentals	Yes	1
	No	2
Relatives	Yes	1
	No	2
Savings withdrawals, sale of real estate, or cashing bonds	Yes	1
	No	2
Other (SPECIFY)	Yes	1
	No	2

15. Is your monthly income over $980?

Yes 1
No 2
Refused to answer.................. 3
N/R 9
(IF NOT MARRIED, SKIP TO
QUESTION 17)

IF MARRIED ASK:

16. Is your monthly income over $1,800 for both you and your spouse?

Yes 1
No 2
N/R 9

17. How long have you lived in this county?

Under 1 year 1
More than 1 but less than 5 years 2
Between 5 and 10 years 3
Longer (SPECIFY) 4
N/R 9

18. What is your present employment status?

Never employed outside the home 1
Full-time work 2
Part-time work 3
Retired 4
N/R 9
(IF NEVER WORKED OR WORKING,
SKIP TO QUESTION 23)

19. At what age did you retire from paid employment?.

Under 60 1
60-64 2
65 3
66-69 4
70-80 5
N/R 9

20. Were you ready for retirement?

Yes 1
No 2
N/R 9
(IF YES, SKIP TO QUESTION 22)

21. IF NO, ASK:

Why not?

(SUGGESTED STANDARD PROBE: For example, did you feel you wanted to continue to work, were you concerned about your income, or was your health involved?)

CIRCLE ALL ANSWERS GIVEN

Enjoyed working	Yes	1
	No	2
Job was whole life	Yes	1
	No	2
Needed the money	Yes	1
	No	2
Deteriorating health	Yes	1
	No	2
Work connected with self-esteem	Yes	1
	No	2
Other (SPECIFY)	Yes	1
	No	2

22. What has been the *MOST* difficult thing about retiring?

Income loss 1
Bored 2
Enjoyed work 3
Feel useless 4
Loss of social contact 5
Other (SPECIFY) 6
N/R 9
(SKIP TO QUESTION 25)

23. Are you satisfied with your present work situation?

Yes 1
No 2
N/R 3
(IF YES, SKIP TO QUESTION 25)

IF NO ASK:

24. Why not?

(SUGGESTED STANDARD PROBE: For example, do you want to change your hours, type of work, income, or would you like to retire?)

Wants to work more hours 1
Wants to work less hours 2
Wants to retire 3
Would like less strenuous work 4
Would like a different type of work 5
N/R 9

25. Comparing yourself to others in your age group and using the following, how would you rate your *health?*
READ THE FOLLOWING:

Much better than others 1
Better than others 2
About the same 3
Worse than others 4
Much worse than others 5
N/R 9

26. What kind of health insurance do you have?
READ LIST AND CIRCLE *ALL* ANSWERS:

Medicare	Yes 1	
	No 2	
Medical	Yes 1	
	No 2	
AARP	Yes 1	
	No 2	
Champus	Yes 1	
	No 2	
Private insurance	Yes 1	
	No 2	
Kaiser	Yes 1	
	No 2	
None	Yes 1	
	No 2	
Other (SPECIFY)	Yes 1	
	No 2	

(IF NONE, SKIP TO QUESTION 28)

27. Does your insurance cover at least one-half of your medical cost?

Yes 1
No 2
Do not know 3
N/R 9

28. How long has it been since you saw a doctor?

Less than 6 months 1
6 months to a year 2
1 to 2 years 3
2 to 5 years 4
Longer (SPECIFY) 5
Never 6
N/R 9

29. If you become totally dependent on others for your care would you prefer to be cared for
    READ LIST

    In a nursing home 1
    At home 2
    Other (SPECIFY) 3
    N/R 9
    (IF NOT AT HOME, SKIP TO
    QUESTION 31)

IF AT HOME, ASK:
30. Who would care for you?
    CIRCLE ALL ANSWERS:

Spouse	Yes 1	
	No 2	
Family	Yes 1	
	No 2	
Friends	Yes 1	
	No 2	
Hired care	Yes 1	
	No 2	
Do not know	Yes 1	
	No 2	
Other (SPECIFY)	Yes 1	
	No 2	

31. No one wants to become totally disabled or to depend completely on others for continuous physical and emotional care. If you became that severely disabled would you want to continue to live?

    Yes 1
    No 2
    Can't make a decision now 3
    Other (SPECIFY) 4

32. Do you have someone (or more than one) in whom you can confide and with whom you can talk over personal problems?

    Yes 1
    No 2
    (IF NO, SKIP TO QUESTION 36)

IF YES, ASK:

33. What relationship is that (or those) person(s) to you?
    CIRCLE *ALL* ANSWERS

Spouse	Yes	1
	No	2
Child	Yes	1
	No	2
Sibling	Yes	1
	No	2
Friend	Yes	1
	No	2
Nurse	Yes	1
	No	2
Doctor	Yes	1
	No	2
Clergyman	Yes	1
	No	2
Social worker	Yes	1
	No	2
Other (SPECIFY)	Yes	1
	No	2

34. Do you feel they are able to give you adequate emotional support when you need it?

Yes	1
No	2
Sometimes	3
N/R	9

(IF YES OR SOMETIMES, SKIP TO
QUESTION 36)

IF NO, ASK:

35. Why not?
    SUGGESTED STANDARD PROBE: For example, do they have the time or the interest or the expertise to assist and support you?
    CIRCLE *ALL* ANSWERS

They are too busy	Yes	1
	No	2
They have family of their own	Yes	1
	No	2
They are not always available	Yes	1
	No	2
They are not always interested	Yes	1
	No	2

They are not able to understand	Yes 1
	No 2
They have too many problems	Yes 1
	No 2
Do not want to burden them	Yes 1
	No 2
Problems are too personal	Yes 1
	No 2
Other (SPECIFY)	Yes 1
	No 2

36. What is your *most* pressing need right now?
CODE ONLY *ONE* ANSWER.

Health care 1
Money 2
Transportation 3
Meals 4
Insurance coverage 5
Counseling 6
Legal assistance 7
Respite 8
Companionship 9
Employment 10
Protection 11
N/R 99

TO EACH RESPONDENT SAY:
Thank you very much for your time and assistance. Your cooperation is greatly appreciated.
We would like to give you a copy of this community resource pamphlet for your use in the future.

SENIOR RESOURCES SURVEY REPORT

Sarah E. Archer, RN, DrPH
Carole D. Kelly, RN, MS
Meladee F. Stankus, RN, BS

Acknowledgments

Ruth Fleshman provided assistance with instrument construction and interviewer training. BS/MS students at the University of California-San Francisco School of Nursing conducted survey interviews:

Amudsen, Marie Nicheole	Kitagawa, Katherine Midori
Armstrong, Sheree Nash	Manny, Sara Mary
Beckes, Anne	Maresca, Joan Gilda
Campbell, Bobbi	Meister, Marleen Lucille
Campbell, Ora Lee	Morrison, Eileen Frances
Carroll, Mary Raenette	Pearce, Melinda Kirk
Collier, Roxena Ruth	Peck, Martha A.
Daniels, Rita Kay	Peirano, Mary Theresa
Desmond, Elizabeth Marie	Pelosi, Patti Kelly
Dickinson, Dena Ethel	Perdew, Debrah Marie
Donker, Patricia Gail	Quinn, Patricia Ann
Freeze, Cynthia Charlene	Schawger, Donna Jean Mc Nine
Gedris, Michele D.	Scott, Peggy R.
Gesulga, Terry A.	Smalstig, Tami D'Ann
Goetz, Constance M.	Swafford, Maria Josephine
Goldmacher, Anna Sue	Szydlowski, Pauline Evelyn
Gomez, Diana S. Castaldi	Thomsen, Andrea Elizabeth
Grey, Susan Patricia	Walker, Nan Victoria
Henry, Marian Frances	Wolfsen, Connie Renee
Hill, Susan L.	

Graduate students supervised the interviews and were responsible for data processing:

Bisch, Sally Ann	Schwartz, Nancy Gail
Eastman, Sharon Snyder	Stankus, Meladee F.
Jung, Mabel Wah	Weber, Gail Gloria
Kelly, Carole Denise	
Luttman, Phyllis A.	
Lynette, Eileen Linda	
McInerney, Katherine Frances	

A study of the county's elderly population conducted for the county Area Agency on Aging by faculty and students for the Department of Mental Health and Community Nursing, School of Nursing, University of California at San Francisco. Survey period: April, May, June, 1981. Report submitted: October, 1981.

Program Directors and staff of the following agencies provided cooperation, interest, and time:

The county college
The county housing authority
The city Multi-Service Center
The county churches
The county libraries
The county newspapers
The Senior Coordinating Council
    Senior information and referral
    Whistlestop junctions
City Human Needs Center
Nursing Dynamics Corporation
    Senior day services
    Senior in-home supportive services project
Senior Citizens' Club
Senior Citizens' Legal Project
Senior Health Project
The Redwoods
Volunteer Bureau

Table of contents

List of tables

List of tables   Page

List of tables   Page

COUNTY AREA AGENCY ON AGING OLDER ADULTS SURVEY
Background

The county Area Agency on Aging is described in its Annual Plan as a planning, coordinating, and grants administration unit within the County Department of Health and Human Services. The agency receives its mandate from the federal Older Americans Act, first passed in 1965. The 1973 amendments to the Act—most of which were products of the concerns voiced by delegates to the 1971 White House Conference on Aging—institutionalized local planning and control through designated Area Agencies on Aging (AAA).

The Older Americans Act carries with it an annual appropriation of federal funds for social and nutrition services for older adults, which are administered by the AAAs. The county's appropriation is sub-contracted to community-based agencies for such programs as transportation, legal services, in-home care, day care, employment, information and referral, and congregate and home-delivered meals.

The AAA was established in 1977 with its main focus on planning and program development to coordinate and pool resources with other public and private organizations to avoid duplication and fragmentation of services and to fund new programs to help meet the needs of older adults in the community.

To meet these goals and to assist in the planning process, public hearings were held. Also, several needs assessments were done. An agency in west county evaluated the services available to older adults in that area to see if the available services met the needs and desires of that population. The AAA requested the same type of evaluation be done for the more densely populated corridor of the county. The study described in this report was undertaken as a joint project by the Health Committee of the county Commission on Aging, a citizen's advisory group to the AAA, and the Department of Mental Health and Community Nursing, School of Nursing, University of California-San Francisco. It served the dual purpose of providing the AAA with the data reported here and offering field experience in community assessment for

graduate and undergraduate students in community health nursing as partial fulfill-
ment of the requirements for several courses.

Purpose

The purpose of this study was to gather information from older adult volunteers
in the county to enable evaluation of their knowledge and use of services available to
people in their age group. The survey instrument is found on pp. 194-205. Since a
study of over 700 elderly had been conducted recently in west county,[5] volunteers
from west county were intentionally excluded from this study. Some of the questions
from the west county survey were included in the interview schedule for this study to
generate comparable data on a county-wide basis.

Methods

Survey subjects were persons over 60 years of age from the county, excluding
residents of those areas included in the west county survey. Participation by subjects
was completely voluntary and confidential. Access to clients posed a major problem,
so the study used a convenience sample. The interviews were conducted by registered nurse students from the University of California-San Francisco School of Nursing during April and May of 1981. The purpose of the study was to determine the use
and knowledge of existing county services as well as to provide for indications of
unmet needs for services in the elderly population of the county. The survey instrument was constructed to facilitate comparison of data with other county surveys.
Specific questions were added, modified, and occasionally eliminated during the
development of the survey instrument. Pretest of the interview schedule by Adult
Day Health Care clients resulted in several subsequent modifications.

The survey data were gathered via interviews because of the length and complexity of the information sought and the sensitive nature of some of the questions.
Another factor that influenced the decision to use an interview was the high incidence of decreased visual acuity in the target population. Additionally, the interview
format lent itself to a useful field experience for students and allowed more in-depth
data to be gathered. The nurse interviewers were trained in interview techniques
using the survey instrument and specific standardized probing methods. The interview time was 1 hour, and each interviewer completed approximately four surveys.

Originally, an attempt was made to gain access to the Social Security lists for the
county so that a systematic random sample of older adults in the corridor area could be
obtained. This was not possible because of confidentiality restrictions on this information. As a result subjects for the study were sought via an invitation to participate
in a number of senior citizens publications as well as in the general press in the
county. Volunteer subjects were asked to call the local senior information and referral
service where their names, addresses, and phone numbers would be recorded by
that agency. The interviewers, who were registered nurses, would then contact the

volunteer to make an appointment to conduct the interview in their home or other mutually convenient place. Because of a variety of factors beyond the control of the investigators, fewer elderly people volunteered than had been hoped. Thus the design had to be modified midstream. This resulted in the survey team soliciting volunteer subjects at a number of sites such as meal sites, congregate housing, and blood pressure clinics.

Limitations

A major constraint of this study involved difficult access to potential survey participants. Limited resources narrowed the options available to approach the access problem. This necessitated that we use a convenience sample. Despite the inclusion of volunteers obtained from groups sites, the total number of subjects surveyed was only 138. These factors limit the representativeness and therefore generalizability of the data reported here. All subjects were self-selected volunteers, a source of bias in the sample. Conjecture is possible that many of the people who responded to media and congregate site invitations to participate in the study were likely to be people who are more aware of and more likely to participate in services available for older adults than were nonvolunteers. Thus the bias resulting from an all-volunteer sample is likely to be in the direction of interviewing people who know more about services and are more, rather than less, involved in them.

Problems of interrater reliability were reduced by interviewer training and supervision. For example, one-sentence descriptions of each service and other standard probes were used by all interviewers. Interviewer training, including a discussion of the interview schedule and role playing, was also conducted. All answer sheets were reviewed immediately after conduct of the interview to reduce the need to delete answers because of recording errors. However, the large number of interviewers used for the study must be assumed to have created some interrater reliability problems, despite this training and supervision.

Findings

Not all respondents answered every question. Thus the "n" or number for each question is different and is indicated each time. The total number of subjects participating in the survey was 138.

Seventy-one subjects (52%) were volunteers. The remaining 67 (48%) participants were solicited from aggregate sites. Participants were fairly equally distributed among southern, central, and northern county.

Demographic characteristics of the survey's subjects. Some of the demographic data from the survey reported here are compared with data for the county as a whole. All county data, unless otherwise specifically cited, are based on 1976 population projections from the California State Department of Finance for July 1, 1980. These data are based on the entire county, including west county; the survey data do not include any data from elderly in west county. The Department of Finance data are used since the 1980 U.S. Census data were not yet available at the time this report was prepared. U.S. Census data for the county before the 1980 Census have not been as detailed as are those reported for standard metropolitan statistical areas. This more detailed reporting of census data is expected to be available from the 1980 census.

Each respondent was asked to indicate her or his residential zip code during the interview. This was the only geographical identifying data obtained. Of the 138 subjects 48 (35%) were from north county, 47 (34%) were from central county, and 43 (31%) were from south county. Thus the participants were evenly distributed geographically on the bayside corridor of the county.

Table 1 shows the distribution of survey respondents by sex, compared with the sex distribution for the county as a whole. The county's proportion of men age 60 and over (44%) exceeds the national average (33%) of men in this age group. In the survey, women over the age of 60 comprise almost three quarters of the respondents. This may be caused at least in part by the selection of aggregate sites where volunteers were sought, that is, congregate meals and subsidized housing.

The sex distribution of respondents in the west county study was 48% male and 52% female; these data show a closer correlation with the overall sex distribution of the 60 and over population in the county than do the data reported here. This may be a reflection of the fact that 60% of the west county respondents were married and living with their spouses, whereas only 34% of the subjects in this study reported similar living arrangements. Table 2 shows the marital status of all of the survey subjects. In addition, only 21% of the west county respondents were widowed compared to 49% widowed in this survey. There are presently no other county-wide data on the marital status of the over-60 population.

Table 3 shows that the majority of women in the sample are widowed, whereas the majority of the men are married and living with their spouses. Again, comparable data are not presently available for the county but have been requested from the 1980 census.

Older women are acknowledged as the elderly majority in this country; this fact is just beginning to be heard at the federal level where program monies are made available. Older women on the whole live longer than men, have less financial income than men, and populate nursing homes at a higher rate than do men. They also become the primary caretakers of their spouses when their husbands become ill. Again, the sample differs slightly from the county data (as shown in Table 4), in that there is a higher percentage of responses from the over-75 age group. This may have to do with the fact that programs are targeted at the older more frail elderly in the population and, since they were a self-selected group, some coming from the program sites themselves, this group may have felt more inclined to respond to the invitation to participate than those who were not involved. In a decision later on knowledge and use of services, please note that 71 respondents were volunteers and 67 came from one of the congregate sites.

TABLE 1

Comparison of senior survey subjects by sex in percentages with
sex distribution in the county (n = 138)

Sex	Sample		County	
	No.	%	No.	%
Male	36	26	13,789	44
Female	102	74	17,550	56

TABLE 2

Marital status of survey subjects by number and by percentages (n = 137)

Marital status	No.	%
Never married	8	6
Separated	2	2
Divorced	13	10
Widowed	67	49
Married, live with spouse	47	34

TABLE 3

Marital status by sex in number and percentages (n = 137)

Marital status	Male		Female	
	No.	%	No.	%
Never married	3	8	5	5
Separated	0	0	2	2
Divorced	3	8	9	9
Widowed	12	32	56	55
Married, living with spouse	19	52	29	29
TOTAL	36	100	102	100

TABLE 4

Ages of subjects in number and percentages (n = 138)

Age in years	Sample		County	
	No.	%	No.	%
60-64	20	14	31,340	75
65-74	66	48		
75-84	37	27	7,859	25
85-106	15	11		
TOTAL	138	100	39,199	100

The county data in Table 3 are of the entire county, although these county data are broken down into rural and urban area totals but not into age or sex categories. An interesting figure that is available for the entire county is that, of the 1799 elderly over the age of 85, 69% are female.

Hispanic/Latino respondents are slightly overrepresented in the study population compared with their proportion of the county's total population, as shown in Table 5.

Income level and income sources of the subjects. The Housing and Urban Development (HUD) Agency's baseline or eligibility income of $980 for a single person and $1800 for a married couple was used as the dividing line for the question about income in this survey. These figures were the ones used to determine qualification for housing assistance in the county area. There were 48 subjects (37%) who indicated that their income was greater than $980. Of those whose income was greater than $980, 42 indicated that this was a combined income with their spouse and that this combined income equaled or exceeded the $1800 identified by HUD.

The data in Table 6 show an almost inverse relationship between sex and income; that is, only 23% of the 95 women respondents have incomes in excess of the HUD criterion, whereas 64% of the 36 men have incomes above these figures. This finding emphasizes the disproportionate numbers of women in low-income brackets.

There were 83 subjects or 63% who have an income of less than $980. Income sources were varied, and many subjects listed several sources. These are shown in Table 7. Social Security was by far the source most frequently given (90%). Seventy-five percent of the respondents in the west county survey indicated that they received Social Security.[5] Investment and interest income ranked second (60%). Less than 1% of the respondents indicated that their relatives provided their income. Many subjects listed more than one source of income.

Retirement. When questioned regarding their current employment status, 136 subjects responded. The majority, 107 (79%) classified themselves as currently retired. Seventy-two percent of the west county sample indicated they were retired.[5] Nineteen subjects in this study (14%) were involved in part-time work outside of the home. Only about 1% of the sample was employed full-time at the time of the survey. Eight respondents (6%) indicated that they had never worked outside of the home.

Table 8 shows that 44% of the survey sample retired at the age of 65 or above. Mandatory retirement is now at the age of 70 and legislation is proposed to remove mandatory retirement age. With the economic restrictions on Social Security suggested by the Reagan administration on retirement before the age of 65, we may see more people working until they are 65 or older. Many people want to continue working as long as they can do so effectively.

All subjects were asked if they had been ready to retire when they did. Of the 115 who responded, 46 (42%) stated that they had not been ready to retire when they did so. Table 9 shows the reasons subjects who were not ready to retire gave for

TABLE 5

Comparison of subjects' ethnic backgrounds by percent
with that of the county (n = 138)

Ethnic make-up	Sample %	County %
White	96	96
Black	1.5	0.5
Hispanic/Latino	1.5	3
Other	1.0	0.5

TABLE 6

Income level by sex, based on Department of Housing and Urban
Development income of $980 per month (n = 131)

	Above $980		Below $980		Total	
Sex	No.	%	No.	%	No.	%
Male	23	64	13	36	36	100
Female	22	23	73	77	95	100

TABLE 7

Income sources of subjects by percentage

Source	%
Social security	90
Interest/investment income	60
Savings bond income	37
Private pension	33
Government pension	30
Income from employment	19
Old age assistance	13
Other	10
Relatives provide income	Less than 1

TABLE 8

Ages of subjects at retirement in number and percentages (n = 116)

Age of retirement	No.	%
under 60	33	28
60-64	33	28
65	18	16
66-69	16	14
70-80	16	14

TABLE 9

Reasons given by 46 subjects who were not ready to retire when they did

Reasons	No.*	%
Enjoyed working	46	100
Needed the money	37	80
Self-esteem through job	36	78
Job was life	10	22
Other reasons	8	17

*Many subjects gave more than one reason.

wanting to continue to work. Over 90% enjoyed their jobs. More than two-thirds saw their jobs as sources of needed income and self-esteem. It is a tragic commentary on our society that people who want to continue to work cannot do so, assuming they are still competent. Recent changes in mandatory retirement legislation will reduce this waste. Although, only 21 subjects (15%) indicated their specific type of current employment, 59 subjects (82%) wanted to work more and 13 (18%) wanted to work less.

These findings are amplified by the data in Table 10, which show the aspects 68 subjects found most difficult for them. The loss of social contact and the loss of income indicated by 52% may account for the high prevalence of loneliness and need for companionship expressed by many retired persons.

Housing. Housing, as is income, is an essential consideration in planning and working with the elderly. Data from 132 subjects in this study show that 49% rented and 51% owned their residence. Six respondents indicated that they neither rented nor owned their living accommodations: two lived with relatives, two were boarders, and two shared a house but declined to disclose the financial arrangements. These findings are very different from those in the west county survey that found 87% of the respondents in that area owned their homes.[5]

Table 11 shows respondent distribution in terms of the people with whom they live. Fifty-eight percent reported that they lived alone; of these 66 (83%) were female. Only 25 percent (169 subjects of the west county participants) reported that they lived alone. That study does not report the sex distribution of those living alone.[5]

Respondents were asked if they were satisfied with their current living arrange-ments. If they indicated that they were not, they were asked what kind they would prefer. Ninety-six subjects (70%) indicated that they were satisfied the way things were. However, 42 said that they would prefer other arrangements; these responses are listed in Table 12. One's own home or apartment are the two leading preferred or ideal housing arrangements given. Sixty (90%) of the respondents in the west county survey indicated that they were comfortable with their living arrangements at the time that survey was conducted.[5] The five subjects who responded "other" did not

TABLE 10
Most difficult aspect of retirement (n = 68)

Aspect	No.	%
Loss of social contact	19	28
Enjoyed work	19	28
Income loss	16	24
Bored	9	13
Felt useless	5	7
TOTAL	75	100

TABLE 11
Persons with whom respondents lived (n = 138)

Living arrangement	No.	%
Alone	80	58
Husband/wife	45	33
Child	8	6
Friend	2	1
Other	3	2
TOTAL	138	100

TABLE 12
Preferred living arrangements (n = 42)

Preferred housing	No.	%
Own home	10	24
Apartment	8	19
Retirement center	6	14
Hotel	5	12
Other	5	12
Sharing housing	3	7
Condominium	3	7
Family home	1	2.5
Board and care home	1	2.5
TOTAL	42	100

indicate what specific kinds of housing they would prefer in lieu of their present situation.

Knowledge of a community depends many times on how long an individual has lived in that community. Table 13 shows that the majority (66%) of those participating in the survey have lived in the county for over 10 years. A small number of respondents (2%) have lived in the county for less than 1 year. Of the respondents to the west county survey, 433 (69%) had lived in the county for more than 10 years at the time they were studied.[5]

Health. Health and the desire to preserve an adequate level of functioning are major concerns for the elderly. It is a fairly generally accepted belief that those people who have maintained their health cope better with stresses and changes that are part of aging than do those whose health has deteriorated. Table 14 shows respondents' self-concept of their own health relative to the health of others their age. Sixty-one percent said that their health was better than others' health, while only 14% said that it was worse. These data are subjective. Each respondent used her or his personal yardstick for comparison purposes. What is important is that those respondents who assess their health as better than or as good as that of others their age are probably more psychologically positive than are those subjects who perceive that their health to be deteriorating more than that of their peers.

The issues of medical care use and health care costs are of great concern to planners and health care providers as well as to the consuming public. Table 15 shows frequent physician use for a group of people, the majority of whom report their health to be better than or at least as good as that of their peers. This is an area for further investigation. Are these physician visits needed? Could the real and perceived benefits of these visits be obtained by other less costly means? Although 97% of the respondents indicated that they had health insurance, they still must make at least partial payment themselves. Unnecessary physician use impacts the total national expenditure for health care. The use of nurses in community and outpatient clinics to monitor and coordinate services and medications could provide high-quality services at reduced costs. Such services are now available to the elderly, but in most cases the physician indicates that the client return to her or him at designated times. Thus the county's plethora of physicians contributes to medical care cost inflation.

The distribution of respondents' medical insurance coverage is presented in Table 16. Many subjects indicated that they had more than one type of medical insurance. Medicare leads the list with 80% of the participants indicating coverage; those not covered by Medicare are the proportion of the sample who had not yet reached the eligibility age at the time that the study was done. Knowledge of the adequacy of one's insurance coverage is vital in light of the high costs of medical care, especially for the elderly. Of the total number of survey respondents, 131 answered the question about their assessment of the adequacy of their medical insurance coverage. The specific question was "Does your medical insurance cover most of your medical care costs?" Of the 131 respondents, 102 (78%) said yes, 20 (15%) said no,

TABLE 13

Length of residence in the county (n = 131)

Length of residence	No.	%
Over 10 years	86	66
5-10 years	17	13
1-5 years	25	19
Less than 1 year	3	2
TOTAL	131	100

TABLE 14

Self-concept of own health (n = 132)

Status	No.	%
Better than others their own age	81	61
Same as others	33	25
Worse than others	14	14
TOTAL	132	100

TABLE 15

Frequency of physician visits (n = 135)

Time frame	No.	%
Within the last 6 months	109	80
6 months-1 year	20	15
Within last 2 years	4	3
2 years or longer	2	2
TOTAL	135	100

TABLE 16

Type of medical insurance coverage (n = 136)

Type of medical insurance	No.*	%
Medicare	108	80
Private insurance	69	51
Medi-cal	26	17
Kaiser	17	13
AARP	12	9
Champus	10	7
None	3	2

*Many respondents had more than one type of medical insurance.

and 9 (7%) did not know. Again this is subjective data in that the definitions of "most" could vary greatly from one respondent to another. However, the data do show that over three quarters of the subjects in this study felt that their insurance did indeed cover most costs, an indication of satisfaction. It is interesting to note that 7% did not know the extent of their medical insurance coverage. The study in west county sought similar data and found that 548 subjects (80%) stated that their medical insurance covered at least one half of their costs.[5]

A major consideration for the elderly in the area of health is the threat of future illness and/or incapacity. For this reason the study addressed the issue of future illness and the kinds of care respondents stated that they would want. These data are essential for planners and community care providers, since much of the responsibility for assuring that the kinds of support service people want to help them with future illness is primarily theirs. Please bear in mind the following three characteristics of the study population when reading this section of the report:

1. Sixty-six percent had incomes below the HUD eligibility level.
2. Fifty-eight percent lived alone.
3. The focus of most health care insurance is on acute institutional care and reimbursement.

On the subject of future illness, the following question was posed: "No one wants to become totally disabled or to depend completely on others for continuous physical or emotional care. If you became severely disabled, would you want to continue to live?" The question was answered by 134 subjects. Thirty-five (26%) said yes, they would want to continue to live, 81 (60%) said no, they would not, and 18 (13%) could not decide at the time of the interview.

Table 17 shows the distribution of subjects' decisions about continuing to live if disabled by age groups. Of the 34 respondents between the ages of 75 and 84 years 8% indicated that they would not wish to continue to live if they were to become disabled, compared to 69% of the 55 subjects aged 65 to 74, and 58% of the 12 subjects aged 85 to 106 who expressed the same desire.

Further examination of the data on desire to live if disabled categorized by respondents' sex is shown in Table 18. Just over one half of the male respondents and almost two thirds of the female respondents indicated that they would not wish to continue to live if disabled. The higher proportion of women who stated that they would not wish to live if disabled could reflect the higher number of women in the sample. Many of the male respondents were already living alone and thus may have realized more clearly how dependent on outside sources of support disability would render them.

Income and marital status are also variables that often influence elderly persons' perceptions of their well-being and so can impact on their desire to continue to live if disabled. Table 19 shows the relationships of the desire of 136 respondents to live if disabled in terms of their marital status and income. The data do not show any marked relationship between the three variables of desire to live, income, and mar-

TABLE 17

Distribution by respondents' age group of desire to continue
to live if disabled (n = 134)

Desire to live	60-64		65-74		75-84		85-106		TOTAL	
	No.	%*	No.	%	No.	%	No.	%	No.	%
Yes	6	4	17	13	7	5	5	4	35	26
No	9	7	38	28	27	20	7	5	81	61
Can not decide now	5	4	8	6	2	1	3	2	18	13
TOTAL	20	15	63	47	36	27	15	11	34	100

*Percentages are of the total of 134.

TABLE 18

Distribution by respondents' sex of desire to
continue to live if disabled (n = 134)

Desire to live	Male		Female	
	No.	%	No.	%
Yes	10	29	25	25
No	18	51	63	64
Cannot decide now	7	20	11	11
TOTAL	35	100	99	100

TABLE 19

Desire to continue to live by marital status and income (n = 136)

Desire to live if disabled	Single				Married				TOTAL	
	<$980		>$980		<1800		>$1800			
	No.	%	No.	%	No.	%	No.	%	No.	%
Yes	22	16	4	3	5	4	2	1	33	24
No	38	28	23	17	11⁻	8	6	5	78	57
Cannot decide now	7	5	11	8	5	4	2	1	25	19
TOTAL	67	49	38	28	21	16	10	7	136	100

ital status, although slightly more than half of the single and married subjects with incomes under the Housing and Urban Development assistance line indicated that they did not wish to continue to live if disabled.

When asked where they would be cared for in the event of a future illness that would render them totally dependent on others for care, almost three quarters of the 134 subjects chose to stay at home. Table 20 shows their responses. Those who said they would want to remain at home were asked to identify the *person* they wanted to care for them. Table 21 shows these data.

The reality is that in most cases the spouse or family provides the care. Given the present reimbursement system for health care services and the level of income for many of the respondents, they would not be able to pay for health care at home for any length of time. Even if they are able to pay, there is a shortage of agencies to provide in-home workers in the county. Given the overwhelming preference subjects in this study stated for hired in-home care, this is a priority that provider agencies and planners need to address.

Support systems. Support systems are important for the maintenance of physical as well as mental health. For the elderly, support systems are an extremely important community component because of the high incidence of illness and crisis situations older people face. For example, loss of a spouse or friends is a frequent occurrence for this age group. This survey addresses both the availability and adequacy of support systems in the county as perceived by the respondents.

Having a confidant—someone with whom one can discuss personal issues openly—is critical for all people. Having a confidant is even more essential for the elderly. Thus respondents were asked if they had someone in whom to confide. Of the total of 138 subjects, 116 (84%) stated that they did have such a person. The three most frequently named persons in terms of the type of relationship they had with the respondents were spouse, friend, and physician. Eighty-four percent of the female respondents and 83% of the male respondents stated that they had someone in whom to confide. Table 22 shows the distribution of various age groups of respondents' reported access to confidants. The table shows that the prevalence of a confidant is extremely high in all age groups and actually increases in the older groups. Length of residence in the county also correlated closely with access to confidants. The longer subjects had lived in the county the more likely they were to have a confidant.

Table 23 shows the distribution of respondents' reported access to a confidant in terms of their marital status. Those subjects who were divorced had the lowest frequency of access to a confidant. Interestingly, those respondents who had never been married had the highest incidence of access to confidants, with married people living with their spouses a close second. Two participants indicated that they were separated; one had a confidant, the other did not. Service providers, particularly community mental health services, must be alert to the needs of those elderly persons who do not have confidants and make their confidant counseling services both known to and available to these members of the community.

TABLE 20
Location of care if severely disabled (n = 134)

Location	No.	%
Home	99	73
Nursing home	23	17
Other	14	10
TOTAL	134	100

TABLE 21
Source of care to respondents who want to be cared for at home (n = 138)

Source of care	No.	%
Hired care	73	70
Family	36	35
Friends	23	22
Spouse	31	30
Do not know	22	24
Other	2	2
TOTAL	138	*

*Total exceeds 100% since many of the respondents gave more than one source for care.

TABLE 22
Distribution of access to confidant by respondents' age group (n = 138)

	Age group							
	60-64		65-74		75-84		85-106	
Have a confidant	No.	%	No.	%	No.	%	No.	%
Yes	16	80	55	83	31	84	14	93
No	4	20	11	17	6	16	1	7
TOTAL	20	100	66	100	37	100	15	100

TABLE 23
Distribution of access to confidant by respondents' marital status (n = 135)

	Never married		Divorced		Widowed		Married, living with spouse	
Have a confidant	No.	%	No.	%	No.	%	No.	%
Yes	7	88	10	77	56	84	41	87
No	1	12	2	23	11	16	6	13
TOTAL	8	100	12	100	72	100	54	100

Subjects were asked if they believed that the support they received from their confidants was adequate. Of the respondents 119 answered the question; 106 (89%) believed that the support they received was adequate, 8 (7%) said sometimes support was adequate, and 5 (4%) said support was inadequate. Specific reasons respondents gave for the inadequacy of the support they received from their confidants were twofold. First, respondents felt that often others did not understand their problems, and second, that they themselves were unwilling to burden other people with their problems. Here again, agencies providing mental health and counseling services to the elderly could help fill the gap.

Needs. Subjects were asked to identify their most pressing need at the time that the interview was conducted. Table 24 shows the responses of 118 participants. Health care leads the list with money and companionship not far behind. Other services needed were insurance coverage, counseling, legal assistance, protection, recreation, shopping assistance, and exercise. Other nonservice needs expressed were time, respect, more cultural activities, and solutions to personal problems.

Comparing the needs expressed by participants in this study with those found by the west county survey shows that the latter group placed better health as their top priority, with home help and transportation tied for second place.[5] Companionship needs between the two groups of respondents were markedly different. Eighteen percent of the participants in the senior resources study reported here listed companionship as their most pressing need; only 5% of the west county respondents so indicated. This discrepancy in need priority can be influenced by several factors: 75% of the west county respondents lived with someone whereas 58% of those in this study lived alone. Furthermore, many people who choose to live in rural areas such as west county do so because they are independent and so rely less on others for support. Finally, the Senior Resources Survey was a self-selected sample, so that the data could be biased by the overrepresentation of people in it who needed companionship and so volunteered to participate. The west county survey was conducted door-to-door.

Knowledge and use of services. Each respondent was asked a series of questions regarding services available for the elderly in the county. A one-sentence description of each service was given as a probe (see questionnaire). These services were divided into two sections; the first was community services and the second was mental health services. The respondents had little difficulty answering the questions regarding knowledge and use, but there was confusion over the other questions. As a result, the questions regarding awareness and use will first be presented from the entire sample. Following that presentation, there will be a comparison to a smaller sample in which all of the questions were answered.

Table 25 lists in rank order the most known services as well as the use by the respondents.

The rank order suggests that those services that focused on generalized long-term community involvement (meal sites through health counseling in Table 25) are

TABLE 24
Respondents' most pressing need (n = 118)

Need	No.	%
Health care	22	19
Money	19	16
Companionship	18	15
Other services	14	12
Transportation	13	11
No pressing need	13	11
Housekeeping	9	8
Respite	6	5
Other	4	3
TOTAL	118	100

TABLE 25
Knowledge and use of services in rank order

Service	Knowledge			Use		
	No.	%	n	No.	%	n
Meal sites	119	86	138	53	43	122
In-home meals	117	85	137	22	18	121
Blood pressure clinic	116	85	137	76	63	120
Transportation	116	84	138	45	38	120
Recreation	116	84	138	61	51	120
Exercise classes	109	81	135	42	37	114
Public health nurse	105	76	138	44	40	110
Senior employment	103	75	137	26	25	106
Legal assistance	100	73	138	46	48	95
Information and referral	89	65	137	46	48	95
Health counseling	88	65	136	49	50	99
Senior health project	86	62	137	42	42	99
Support services from churches	84	62	135	43	46	94
Day care for the elderly	81	59	137	7	7	95
In-home services	74	54	136	21	24	89
Friendly visitors	53	39	135	13	19	70
Outreach	48	36	134	19	29	65
Nursing home ombudsman	37	28	133	5	9	55
Adult protective services	23	17	134	7	14	52

the most widely known. The second grouping (senior health project through friendly visitors) are personal and individual sevices and are not quite as well known. The last three (outreach, ombudsman, and protective services) are more specialized and so are least well known. Knowledge of the services of Information and Referral was indicated by only 65% of the subjects; since 52% of the sample called Information and Referral to volunteer to participate in the survey, one might assume that they knew something of its services. If that is true, than only 13% of the sample that was obtained from the congregate sites had knowledge of Information and Referral's services. This seems implausible. One possible explanation for the low reported knowledge of Information and Referral service might be that consumers do not give the same title to programs as do providers. However, if an agency's purpose is to provide a specific type of service, perhaps there is a need to clarify the nature of that service so that it is readily understood by potential consumers.

Use of services fell into a different rank order than did the knowledge of services. Table 26 shows the rank ordering of respondents' use of services. The most heavily used services such as blood pressure clinics and recreation are those that are accessible to the more mobile members of the community; those services aimed at the less mobile, for example nursing home ombudsman and adult day care, are understandably less used by members of the respondent group.

When the sample is divided into volunteer and congregate site participants, some differences in awareness of services become apparent. Table 27 and 28 show the rank ordering of the knowledge of these services by volunteer and congregate site participants.

TABLE 26
Respondents' use of services in rank order

Service	Use (%)
Blood pressure clinic	63
Recreation	51
Health counseling	50
Legal assistance	48
Information and referral	48
Support services from churches	46
Meal sites	43
Senior health project	42
Public health nurse	40
Transportation	38
Exercise classes	37
Outreach	29
Senior employment	25
In-home services	24
Friendly visitors	19
In-home meals	18
Adult protective services	14
Nursing home ombudsman	9
Day care for the elderly	7

TABLE 27

Rank order of knowledge of services demonstrated by volunteer
participants (n = 71)

Service	Knowledge (%)
Recreation	87
In-home meals	86
Meal site	85
Transportation	85
Blood pressure clinic	80
Exercise	79
Public health nurse	78
Senior employment	73
Legal assistance	70
Support services (church)	70
Health counseling	61
Senior health project	59
Information and referral	58
Day care	57
In-home services	57
Outreach	36
Friendly visitors	35
Nursing home ombudsman	24
Adult protective services	19

TABLE 28

Rank order of knowledge of services demonstrated by congregate site
participants (n =67)

Service	Knowledge (%)
Blood pressure clinic	91
Meal site	90
Transportation	88
In-home meals	88
Recreation	87
Exercise	84
Public health nurse	79
Senior employment	78
Legal assistance	74
Information and referral	71
Health counseling	70
Senior health project	66
Day care	63
Support services (church)	58
In-home services	54
Friendly visitors	42
Outreach	36
Nursing home ombudsman	31
Adult protective services	16

Volunteer participants had greater awareness of:
1. Support services from churches by 12%
2. In-home services by 3%
3. Adult protective services by 3%

Congregate respondents had greater awareness of:
1. Blood pressure clinics by 11%
2. Health counseling by 9%
3. Senior health protective by 7%
4. Nursing home ombudsman by 6%
   Friendly visitors by 6%
   Day care by 6%
5. Senior employment by 5%
   Meal sites by 5%
   Exercise by 5%
6. Legal assistance by 4%
7. Information and referral by 3%
   Transportation by 3%
8. In-home meals by 2%

The remaining three services (Outreach, Public health nurse, and Recreation) were within 1% of each other.

Table 29 indicates the levels of knowledge and use of mental health services demonstrated by 115 respondents. Mental health services are generally underused by the elderly. This sample shows further that the elderly do not acknowledge much familiarity with the mental health services. There may be several reasons for this. Mental health and related therapies are relatively new and therefore are not part of the older person's social support system. Second, in this age group there is a cultural stigma attached to psychiatric problems. This is lessening with time but still has its impact on the use of services by the elderly. Third, and very importantly, is the lack of realization by service providers such as physicians that mental health services are a

TABLE 29
Knowledge and use of mental health services in rank order (n = 115)

Service	Knowledge		Use	
	No.	%	No.	%
Crisis unit	48	42	1	.8
Outpatient unit	34	30	1	.8
Companion program	32	28	0	0
Home visits for older adults	26	23	3	3
Developmental disabilities unit	19	17	0	0
Transitional services	17	15	0	0
Mobile geriatric evaluation team	14	12	3	3

viable source of help for the older person. When there is a change in the above three reasons for not using services, the elderly may begin to take advantage of them.

Subset analysis. The following tables and discussion are on a subset of respondents from whom indepth data are available. The levels of awareness and use of services by this group are within 1% of the awareness and use levels of the entire sample of 138 reported in Table 25. Not all of the respondents in this subset provided information on all of the services; thus the number of respondents about any given service may vary.

In the following tables, data for each service are presented separately. In columns three and six only the most prevalent reasons for nonuse are given. The services' tables are presented in descending order of respondents' awareness.

TABLE 30
Knowledge and use of recreation services (n = 81)

Response	Are you aware of this?	Have you used it?	If no, why not?	Do you know others who have used it?	Would you use it if needed?	If no, why not?
Yes	71	39	—	45	52	—
No	10	32	13*	20	9	4*

*Not needed. Even when asked if this service would be used if needed, some respondents felt it would not.

TABLE 31
Knowledge and use of meal sites (n = 81)

Response	Are you aware of this?	Have you used it?	If no, why not?	Do you know others who have used it?	Would you use it if needed?	If no, why not?
Yes	71	35	—	45	55	—
No	10	36	26*	20	7	2†
						2‡

*Not needed.
†Not interested.
‡Have private resources.

TABLE 32
Knowledge and use of transportation services (n = 81)

Response	Are you aware of this?	Have you used it?	If no, why not?	Do you know others who have used it?	Would you use it if needed?	If no, why not?
Yes	70	26	—	46	54	—
No	11	44	32*	18	5	2†

*Not needed.
†Have private resources.

TABLE 33
Knowledge and use of in-home meals (n = 79)

Response	Are you aware of this?	Have you used it?	If no, why not?	Do you know others who have used it?	Would you use it if needed?	If no, why not?
Yes	67	15	—	24	51	—
No	12	52	48* 1†	13	12	1* 2‡

*Not needed.
†Not interested.
‡Have private resources.

TABLE 34
Knowledge and use of public health nursing services (n = 81)

Response	Are you aware of this?	Have you used it?	If no, why not?	Do you know others who have used it?	Would you use it if needed?	If no, why not?
Yes	63	24	—	28	50	—
No	18	37	33*	30	8	1* 1† 2‡

*Not needed.
†Not interested.
‡Have private resources.

TABLE 35
Knowledge and use of legal assistance (n = 81)

Response	Are you aware of this?	Have you used it?	If no, why not?	Do you know others who have used it?	Would you use it if needed?	If no, why not?
Yes	59	18	—	21	43	—
No	22	41	31* 7†	32	7	2†

*Not needed.
†Have private resources. The other response to column 6 was that legal assistance could not help with their specific problem.

TABLE 36
Knowledge and use of senior employment (n = 81)

Response	Are you aware of this?	Have you used it?	If no, why not?	Do you know others who have used it?	Would you use it if needed?	If no, why not?
Yes	58	11	—	24	39	—
No	23	47	24*	13	12	1*
			11†			5†
			4‡			1‡
			7§			1§
						4‖

*Not needed.
†Not interested.
‡Too ill.
§Have private resources.
‖No transportation. Three interesting responses to the last column were didn't like the type of work offered, couldn't exceed SSI requirements, and didn't want to work anymore.

TABLE 37
Knowledge and use of support services from churches (n = 81)

Response	Are you aware of this?	Have you used it?	If no, why not?	Do you know others who have used it?	Would you use it if needed?	If no, why not?
Yes	55	29	—	31	38	—
No	26	26	18*	23	5	1*
			3† 1‡			

Support services were not used by some because they were not church affiliated. This then is not an option available to everyone.
*Not needed.
†Not interested.
‡No transportation.

TABLE 38
Knowledge and use of senior health project (n = 81)

Response	Are you aware of this?	Have you used it?	If no, why not?	Do you know others who have used it?	Would you use it if needed?	If no, why not?
Yes	54	28	—	31	35	—
No	27	26	14*	20	7	1†
			1†			4‡
			8‡			
			3§			

*Not needed.
†Not interested.
‡No transportation.
§Have private resources. An interesting comment about not using the service was that the personal physician did not like it.

TABLE 39
Knowledge and use of health counseling (n = 81)

Response	Are you aware of this?	Have you used it?	If no, why not?	Do you know others who have used it?	Would you use it if needed?	If no, why not?
Yes	54	28	—	30	37	—
No	27	26	19* 1† 1‡ 5§	19	6	4* 2†

*Not needed.
†Not interested.
‡Too ill.
§Have private resources.

TABLE 40
Knowledge and use of Information and Referral (n = 81)

Response	Are you aware of this?	Have you used it?	If no, why not?	Do you know others who have used it?	Would you use it if needed?	If no, why not?
Yes	51	29	—	22	38	—
No	30	22	19* 2† 1‡	23	1	1*

This service was referred to in the larger sample. There is some concern over whether or not there is a confusing factor that Information and Referral is known by its agency name instead of the service. The probe that described the service should have clarified that to the respondents.
*Not needed.
†Not interested.
‡Have private resources.

TABLE 41
Knowledge and use of in-home services (n = 80)

Response	Are you aware of this?	Have you used it?	If no, why not?	Do you know others who have used it?	Would you use it if needed?	If no, why not?
Yes	84	9	—	37	43	—
No	32	39	4* 1†	15	2	1* 1†

*Not needed.
†Too ill.

TABLE 42
Knowledge and use of day care for the elderly (n = 81)

Response	Are you aware of this?	Have you used it?	If no, why not?	Do you know others who have used it?	Would you use it if needed?	If no, why not?
Yes	46	2	—	16	40	—
No	35	44	4* 3† 4‡	28	3	1* 2† 1§

*Not needed.
†Not interested.
‡Too ill.
§No transportation.

TABLE 43
Knowledge and use of friendly visitors (n = 81)

Response	Are you aware of this?	Have you used it?	If no, why not?	Do you know others who have used it?	Would you use it if needed?	If no, why not?
Yes	30	5	—	10	21	—
No	51	25	23* 2†	18	5	2* 2†

*Not needed.
†Not interested.

TABLE 44
Knowledge and use of outreach service (n = 81)

Response	Are you aware of this?	Have you used it?	If no, why not?	Do you know others who have used it?	Would you use it if needed?	If no, why not?
Yes	27	8	—	13	23	—
No	54	19	18* 1†	12	2	1†

*Not interested.
†Not needed. One response as to why they wouldn't use it was that they heard that it wasn't being refunded.

TABLE 45
Knowledge and use of nursing home ombudsman (n = 81)

Response	Are you aware of this?	Have you used it?	If no, why not?	Do you know others who have used it?	Would you use it if needed?	If no, why not?
Yes	21	2	—	9	18	—
No	60	19	17* 11†	12	2	2*

*Not needed.
†Not interested.

TABLE 46
Knowledge and use of adult protective services (n = 81)

Response	Are you aware of this?	Have you used it?	If no, why not?	Do you know others who have used it?	Would you use it if needed?	If no, why not?
Yes	19	6	—	7	17*	—
No	62	13	11*	12	0	0

Note that though this service was the least known, it was accepted by a large majority for future use.
*Not needed.

Respondents who indicated that they knew about programs and services that the survey addressed, were asked about their future use of those programs and services should they need them. As shown in Table 47, the majority of their responses about future of programs and services was positive.

In-home services rank highest in this table of projected future usage of services. This finding is congruent with the high emphasis respondents placed on their desires to remain at home even if disabled. The high projected usage of friendly visitors, support services from churches, and in-home meals are also consistent with the desire to be maintained at home.

Certain factors must be borne in mind when considering the data in the previous tables about awareness and projected use of services and programs. First of all, the data are based on a very small, self-selected sample. Secondly, one must wonder what realistic thought respondents have really given to their future needs and desires. Many changes in life come as a result of crisis situations, situations to which the elderly are particularly prone. Some individuals may have a great deal of difficulty imagining now what services and programs they may need in the future. For example, one of the largest programs on the basis of nationwide need under the Older Americans' Act is nutrition. Yet, the future use of nutrition programs was ranked

TABLE 47

Respondents' awareness and projections of future
use of services and programs (n = 81)

Service or program	Number aware of service or program	Number who would use service or program, if needed	Percentage who would use service or programs, if needed (%)
In-home services	48	43	90
Nursing home ombudsman	19	17	89
Friendly visitors	46	40	86
Outreach	21	18	86
Support services from churches	27	23	85
In-home meals	69	41	80
Senior employment	63	50	79
Legal assistance	71	55	77
Transportation	70	54	77
Adult protective services	30	23	76
Exercise classes	51	38	74
Information and referral	71	52	73
Senior health project	55	38	70
Health counseling	54	37	68
Recreation	59	43	67
Blood pressure clinic	58	39	67
Day care for the elderly	69	42	60
Meal sites	69	41	59

lowest by subjects in this survey. People use services and programs only when the need actually arises.

Mental health services: knowledge and use. As discussed earlier, mental health service use by the elderly is lower than their proportion of the populations would lead one to expect, for a variety of reasons. The following tables show the responses of 115 participants who answered the questions dealing with these programs and services. The tables are in descending order of respondent awareness.

TABLE 48
Knowledge and use of crisis unit (n = 115)

Response	Are you aware of this?	Have you used it?	If no, why not?	Do you know others who have used it?	Would you use it if needed?	If no, why not?
Yes	48	1	—	15	39	—
No	67	114	44* 61†	100	76	1* 3†

*Not needed.
†Have private resources.

TABLE 49
Knowledge and use of outpatient mental health units (n = 115)

Response	Are you aware of this?	Have you used it?	If no, why not?	Do you know others who have used it?	Would you use it if needed?	If no, why not?
Yes	34	1	—	15	39	—
No	81	114	1*	100	76	1* 3†

*Not interested.
†Have private resources.

TABLE 50
Knowledge and use of mental health companion program (n = 115)

Response	Are you aware of this?	Have you used it?	If no, why not?	Do you know others who have used it?	Would you use it if needed?	If no, why not?
Yes	32	0	—	9	44	—
No	83	115	31* 1†	106	71	1*, 1† 3‡

*Not needed.
†Not interested.
‡Have private resources.

TABLE 51
Knowledge and use of mental health home visits for older adults (n = 115)

Response	Are you aware of this?	Have you used it?	If no, why not?	Do you know others who have used it?	Would you use it if needed?	If no, why not?
Yes	26	3	—	9	19	—
No	89	112	19*	106	96	1* 1†

*Not needed.
†Have private resources.

TABLE 52
Knowledge and use of mental health services for persons
with developmental disabilities (n = 115)

Response	Are you aware of this?	Have you used it?	If no, why not?	Do you know others who have used it?	Would you use it if needed?	If no, why not?
Yes	19	0	—	7	14	—
No	96	115	19*	108	111	1* 1†

*Not needed.
†Have private resources.

TABLE 53
Knowledge and use of mental health transitional services (n = 115)

Response	Are you aware of this?	Have you used it?	If no, why not?	Do you know others who have used it?	Would you use it if needed?	If no, why not?
Yes	17	0	—	18	14	—
No	98	115	15*	107	101	0

*Not needed.

TABLE 54
Knowledge and use of mental health mobile geriatric evaluation team (n = 115)

Response	Are you aware of this?	Have you used it?	If no, why not?	Do you know others who have used it?	Would you use it if needed?	If no, why not?
Yes	14	0	—	3	8	—
No	101	115	14*	112	107	1* 1†

*Not needed.
†Have private resources.

TABLE 55

Respondents' awareness and projections of future use of mental health
services and programs (n = 115)

Service or program	Number aware of service or program	Number who would use service or program, if needed	Percentage who would use service or program, if needed (%)
Mobile geriatric evaluation team	17	14	82
Crisis unit	48	39	81
Transition services	32	24	75
Home visits for older adults	14	8	75
Developmental disabilities	19	14	74
Outpatient services	34	25	73
Companion program	26	19	73

The most startling finding in the tables concerning knowledge and use of mental health services by the elderly participants in this study is the lack of information about these services. The vast majority of respondents indicated that they did not know that this array of mental health services has been made available to them. It is encouraging to note, however, that many subjects who knew of the mental health services indicated that they would use them if necessary.

Table 55 shows the percentage of those who are aware of the mental health services who indicate that they would use those services in the future, if needed. Services and programs are listed in descending order of the percentage of those who are aware of them and would use them if needed. As can be seen in the table, the data are from a very small number of respondents. However, the uniformly high percentage of those who are aware of the services and programs and who would use them if needed should be encouraging to those in the mental health area.

Recommendations

Generally increased awareness of services raises the probability of higher future use. Many of the services and programs included in this survey were and are operating at full capacity given their current resources. The ramifications of federal and state budget cuts and deficits are still not completely apparent at the time of this writing (October 1981). It seems safe to say, however, that short of major alternative sources of funding in large amounts becoming available to many of the study's target services, little future expansion is likely. Thus to create greater demand for these services by strategies designed to increase their visibility and acceptability to potential clients is self-defeating when long waiting lists and turnaways are already agencies' and potential clients' problems.

Given that caveat, the survey team believes that the following recommendations warrant consideration.

1. There appears to be a need for pre-retirement planning. Given that 58, or 42%, of the subjects asked were not ready for retirement, some focus should be put on preparing individuals for that part of their lives. This would include second career and increased part-time work options.

2. Consumer education, perhaps as part of the pre-retirement counseling, needs to address the coverage of Medicare and other insurances as contrasted with current medical expenses. This will help people to better understand the strengths and limitations of their coverage. Furthermore, the desire to be cared for at home in the event of a disabling future illness is seen by the respondents as a high priority, and the caregiver would be a hired person, not a spouse or family member. Given reimbursement patterns of most insurance and the limited availability of appropriate personnel to hire for home care, this option does not appear to be possible for many of the subjects who indicated this choice. Changes in insurance coverage along these lines need to be addressed.

3. Programs that emphasize health would apear to be resources since health was identified as the most pressing need. Public health nursing and exercise fall into that category.

4. Opportunities for employment is needed since 113, or 82%, of the subjects were not happy with their work status and would like more work. Many felt that jobs they had been referred to through existing employment services were meaningless and unattractive.

5. Education about available mental health services is crucial. There is a lack of mental health awareness and the need for education of potential consumers, families, and particularly providers of health services (e.g., physicians) is essential. A strong liaison beteen the community mental health programs and the AAA could begin to bridge the gap and serve as a powerful force in the direction of making mental health services more widely known, accepted, and used.

6. Evaluation of the use of physician services should be done to see if these services are appropriate. In light of the fact that the majority of the respondents felt they were in better health than the average, one questions if frequent doctor visits are appropriate. Perhaps other kinds of services such as those of nurse practitioners could better meet their needs.

7. More comparable data are necessary but since the AAA is only three years old there has been limited time to create a needed data base. It is the understanding of this team that more detailed data have been requested from the 1980 Census by the AAA staff. This will assist planners and programers enormously in the future. Another source of data on area elderly can be found in the

Nursing Dynamics Corporation–University of California at San Francisco study of elderly in four north bay counties.[6]

8. There appears to be considerable confusion on respondents' parts about the specific aims and purposes of many of the services and programs targeted in this study. Programs and services need to be clearly defined so that real and potential users understand them. This can be a particular problem for multi-service agencies, but does not lessen the need for community education.

9. There is a need for future studies. This survey only scratches the surface and was extremely limited in its scope and sample. The built-in bias associated with self-selected sample has been discussed. There is a real need to get out into the community on a door to door basis and speak with the elderly in the county. Only then will a true picture of the total elderly population evolve and will the needs of an entire community be adequately assessed. This is an extremely expensive and time-consuming enterprise.

DEPARTMENT OF HEALTH AND HUMAN SERVICES
AREA AGENCY ON AGING
SENIOR RESOURCES SURVEY*
EXECUTIVE SUMMARY
Prepared by Lynn Friss

Purpose

The purpose of the study was to gather information from older persons to determine their knowledge and use of existing services in the county as well as to provide for indications of unmet needs in the county's older population.

Methods and limitations

Due to sampling limitations, a convenience sample was utilized made up of self-selected volunteers, a source of bias in the study.

A total of 138 persons 60 years and older residing in the north, south, and central county were interviewed. Since a study of older residents in the west county had recently been undertaken by the west county senior services, persons from this geographical area were intentionally excluded from this study.

Initially, survey participants were sought through advertisements in a number of senior citizen publications as well as the general press in the county. Volunteers were asked to call the Senior I & R Project in the county and leave their names, addresses, and phone numbers if they would like to participate in the survey. Because fewer

*A 1981 study of a sample of the county's older population conducted by faculty and students of the Department of Mental Health and Community Nursing, School of Nursing, University of California, San Francisco.

persons volunteered than had been hoped for, the survey team solicited participants from a number of community sites in the county such as dining sites, congregate housing, and blood pressure clinics.

Interviews—taking approximately one hour to administer—were conducted by registered nurse students from the UCSF School of Nursing during April and May of 1981. The survey instrument (i.e., interview schedule) was constructed to facilitate comparison of data with the west county survey.

A major constraint of this study involved access to potential survey participants. Limited resources narrowed the options available to approach the sampling problem. All of the respondents were self-selected volunteers. Thus the bias resulting from an all-volunteer sample is likely to be in the direction of interviewing people who know more about services and are more, rather than less, involved in them.

Findings

Among the most significant findings are the following:

Demographic characteristics

Of the 138 respondents, 35 percent (48) were from north county, 34 percent (47) were from central county, and 31 percent (43) were from south county.

The majority of the women surveyed (56 persons or 55 percent) were widowed, while the majority of the men (19 or 52 percent) were married and living with their spouses. Nationally, 56 percent of older women are widowed.

Almost 40 percent of the sample was over 75 years of age (52 persons, 38 percent) compared to about 25 percent of the older population 75+ in the county as a whole.

Income

Of those responding, 77 percent (73) of the women had incomes below the Department of Housing and Urban Development's eligibility income of $980 per month, as compared with only 36 percent (13) of the men. This emphasizes the disproportionate numbers of women in low-income brackets.

Retirement

Regarding retirement, 42 percent (46) of the respondents stated that they had not been ready to retire when they did so.

Housing

Fifty-one percent of the sample owned their residence and 49 percent rented. For the county as a whole, 70 percent of older pesons are homeowners as compared to 30 percent who are renters (1970 census data).

In terms of living arrangement, more than half (58 percent) of the sample lived alone. One-third lived with a spouse, 6 percent lived with a child, 1 percent lived with a friend and 2% had other living arrangements.

Two thirds of the sample lived in the county for over 10 years. A small number of respondents (2 percent), lived in the county for less than one year.

Health

Sixty-one percent of the respondents said their health was better than others
their own age, while only 14 percent said that it was worse. The remaining
25 percent said their health status was the same as others their age.

Despite the majority who reported their health to be better than or at least as
good as that of their peers' health, 80 percent showed frequent physician
utiliation—or a visit within the last 6 months.

When asked where they would like to be cared for in the event of a future illness
that would render them totally dependent on others for care, almost three
quarters (73 percent) of the respondents chose to stay at home. Seventeen
percent chose a nursing home, and another 10 percent chose other living
arrangements.

Support systems

Respondents were asked if they had someone in whom to confide. Eighty-four
percent of the sample stated that they did have such a person. The three
most frequently mentioned confidants were spouse, friend, and physician.
Moreover, the longer the respondent had lived in the county, the more
likely they were to have a confidant.

Needs

Respondents were asked to identify their most pressing need at the time that the
interview was conducted. The top three needs mentioned—comprising 50
percent of the responses—were health care, income, and companionship.

Knowledge and use of services

Those services which focused on generalized long-term community involvement
(e.g., nutrition project, blood pressure clinics, transportation, recreation,
exercise clinics, legal assistance) were the most widely known. The second
grouping (e.g., support services from churches, day care, in-home services,
and friendly visitors) are personal and individualized services and were not
quite as well known. The last grouping comprised of outreach, ombudsman
and protective services are the most specialized and so were the least well
known.

Knowledge of Information and Referral (I&R) services was indicated by only 65
percent of the respondents. Moreover, only 13 percent of the congregate
dining site sample had knowledge of I&R's services. While 65 percent had
knowledge of the service, less than half (48 percent) actually utilized I&R.

While 86 percent of the sample had knowledge of dining sites, less than half (43
percent) used the program.

The most utilized services (e.g., blood pressure clinics and recreation) were
found to be those services that are accessible to more mobile persons. While
the least utilized services (e.g., Ombudsman and adult protective services)

were found to be those services targeted to a smaller and more frail segment of the older population.

Future service use

In-home services ranked highest in projected future usage of services. This finding is congruent with the high emphasis respondents placed on their desire to remain at home even if disabled. The high projected usage of friendly visitors, support services from churches, and in-home meals are also consistent with the desire to remain at home.

Adult day care and congregate dining sites ranked lowest in projected future usage of services. While the relatively low response to projected use of day care can be attributed to a lack of education about the program's benefits, it is unclear why the future use of the congregate nutrition program was ranked lowest when the respondents had the most knowledge of this program.

Recommendations

There appears to be a need for pre-retirement planning. Given that 42 percent of the respondents were not ready for retirement, some focus should be placed on preparing individuals for that part of their lives, including second career and part-time options.

Additionally, expanded opportunities for employment is suggested since 82 percent of those sampled were not happy with their work status and would like more employment opportunities. Many felt that jobs they had been referred to through existing employment services were meaningless and unattractive.

Education about available mental health services is needed. There is a lack of mental health awareness and the need for education of potential consumers, families, and particularly providers of health services (e.g., physicians) is essential. While about 2-5 percent of the older population utilizes mental health services, the need for such services is estimated to range from 15 to 25 percent of the population 65 years and older.

There appears to be considerable confusion—expressed by respondents—about the specific aims and purposes of many of the services and programs targeted in this study. Programs and services need to be clearly defined so that real and potential users understand them. This can be a particular problem for multi-service agencies, but does not lessen the need for community education.

There is a need for future needs assessment surveys. This study only scratched the surface and was limited in its scope and sample. There is a real need to get out into the community on a door-to-door basis and speak with the elderly in the county. Only then will a true picture of the total older population evolve and the needs of an entire community be adequately assessed.

REFERENCES

1. Archer, S.E., and Fleshman, R.P.: Faculty role modeling: opportunities presented by Nursing Dynamics Corporation, Nursing Outlook **29:**586-589, October 1981.
2. Babbie, E.R.: Survey research methods, Belmont, Calif., 1973, Wadsworth Publishing Co., Inc.
3. Bulbul, P.I.: Everybody's studying us: ironies of aging in the Pepsi generation, San Francisco, 1976, Glide Publication.
4. Nie, N.H., and others: Statistical package for the social sciences, ed. 2, New York, 1975, McGraw-Hill Book Co.
5. Growing Old in the Country, Survey performed by West County Senior Services, 1981.
6. Archer, S.E., and others: Life-style indicators for interventions to facilitate elderly persons' independence, Health values: achieving high level wellness 3(3):129-135, 1979.

GENERAL
BIBLIOGRAPHY

Ackoff, R.: Toward a system of systems concepts, Management Science **17**:661-671, July 1971.

Ackoff, R.: Redesigning the future, New York, 1974, John Wiley & Sons, Inc.

Alinsky, S.: Rules for radicals: a pragmatic primer for realistic radicals, New York, 1971, Vintage Books.

Allport, G.W.: The open system in personality theory, Journal of Abnormal and Social Psychology **61**:301-310, November 1960.

Altshuler, A.: Community control, New York, 1970, The Bobbs-Merrill Co., Inc.

Anderson, J.E.: Public policy-making, New York, 1975, Praeger Publishers, Inc.

Andrews, F.M.: Social indicators of perceived quality of life, Social Indicators Research **1**:270-299, 1974.

Archer, S.E., and Fleshman, R.P.: Community health nursing: patterns and practice, ed. 2, N. Scituate, Mass., 1979, Duxbury Press.

Archer, S.E., and Goehner, P.: Nurses: a political force, Belmont, Calif., 1982, Wadsworth Publishing Co., Inc.

Argyres, C.: Intervention theory and method, Reading, Mass., 1970, Addison-Wesley Publishing Co., Inc.

Ashby, W.R.: Design for a brain: the origin of adaptive behavior, London, 1960, Chapman and Hall, Ltd.

Ashby, W.R.: An introduction to cybernetics, London, 1964, Metheun & Co., Ltd.

Ashworth, P.: The role of the clinical nurse consultant, Nursing Mirror **142**:46-48, 1976.

Babbie, E.E.: Survey research methods, Belmont, Calif., 1973, Wadsworth Publishing Co., Inc.

Baizerman, M., and Hall, W.T.: Consultation as a political process, Community Mental Health Journal **13**(2):142-149, Summer 1977.

Baker, J.K., and Schoffer, R.N.: Making staff consulting more effective, Harvard Business Review, January-February, 1979, pp. 62-71.

Bauer, R.: Social indicators, Cambridge, Mass., 1966, The M.I.T. Press.

Beckhard, R.: Helping a group with planned change: a case study, The Journal of Social Issues **15**:13-19, 1959.

Beisser, A., and Green, R.: Mental health consultation and education, Palo Alto, Calif., 1972, National Press Books.

Benne, K.D.: Some ethical problems in group and organizational consultation, The Journal of Social Issues **15**:60-67, 1959. (Also reprinted in Bennis, W., et al., 1976.)

Bennis, W., and others: The planning of change, ed. 3, New York, 1976, Holt, Rinehart & Winston, Inc.

Biddle, W., and Biddle, L.: The community development process, New York, 1965, Holt, Rinehart & Winston, Inc.

Blake, R.R., and Morton, J.S.: Consultation, Reading, Mass., 1976, Addison-Wesley Publishing Co., Inc.

Block, P.: Flawless consulting: a guide to getting your expertise used, San Diego, Calif., 1981, University Associates.

Blum, H.: Planning for health: development and application of social change theory, New York, 1974, Behavioral Publications, Inc.

Blum, H.: Expanding health care horizons: from a general systems concept of health to a national health policy, Oakland, Calif., 1976, Third Party Associates.

Blum, H.: Planning for health, New York, 1978, Human Sciences Press.

Blumberg, A.: A selected annotated bibliography on the consultant relationship with groups, Journal of Social Issues **15**:68-74, 1959.

Braden, C., and Herbon, N.: Community health: a systems approach, New York, 1976, Appleton-Century-Crofts.

Brager, G., and Specht, H.: Community organizing, New York, 1973, Columbia University Press.

Brusegard, D.A., Social indicators 1976, and Perspective Canada II: Elixirs of reason or of sleep? Annals of the American Academy of Political and Social Science **435**:268-276, 1978.

Buckley, W.: Sociology and modern systems theory, Englewood Cliffs, N.J., 1967, Prentice-Hall, Inc.

Bull, N.: Team work, working together in human services, Philadelphia, 1976, J.B. Lippincott Co.

Campbell, D.T.: Focal local indicators for social program evaluation, Social Indicators Research **3**:237-256.

Caplan, G.: Principles of preventative psychiatry, New York, 1964, Basic Books, Inc., Publishers.

Caplan, G.: The theory and practice of mental health consultation, New York, 1970, Basic Books Inc., Publishers.

Caplan, N., and Barton, E.: Social indicators 1973: a study of the relationship between the power of information and utilization by federal executives, Ann Arbor, Mich., 1976, Institute for Social Research, University of Michigan.

Carmichael, N., and Parke, R.: Information services for social indicators research, Special Libraries **65**:209-215.

Chen, M.M., Bush, J.W., and Patrick, D.L.: Social indicators for health planning and policy analysis, Policy Sciences **6**:71-89.

Churchman, C.W.: The systems approach, New York, 1968, Dell Publishing Co., Inc.

Churchman, C.W.: Design of inquiring systems, New York, 1979, Basic Books Inc., Publishers.

Clark, T.N.: Community social indicators: from analytical models to policy applications, Urban Affairs Quarterly **9**:3-36, 1973.

Claus, K.E., and Bailey, J.T.: Facilitating change: a problem solving/decisionmaking tool, Nursing Leadership **2**:30-39, 1979.

Cox, F., and others: Strategies of community organization: a book of readings, ed. 2, Itasca, Ill., 1974, F.E. Peacock Publishers, Inc.

D'Agostino, R.B.: Social indicators: a statistician's view, Social Indicators Research **1**:459-484, 1975.

Deloughery, G., and Gebbie, K.: Political dynamics: impact on nurses and nursing, St. Louis, 1975, The C.V. Mosby Co.

Deloughery, G., Gebbie, K., and Newman, B.: Consultation and community organization in community mental health nursing, Baltimore, 1971, The Williams & Wilkins Co.

Dever, G.: Community health analysis: a holistic approach, Germantown, Md., 1980, Aspen Systems Corp.

Duffus, R.: Lillian Wald: neighbor and crusader, New York, 1938, Macmillan, Inc.

Durbin, R.L., and Springall, W.H.: Organization and administration of health care: theory, practice, environment, ed. 2, St. Louis, 1974, The C.V. Mosby Co.

Dylag, H.: The consultation matrix in community mental health. In Hall, J., and Weaver, B., editors: Distributive nursing practice: a systems approach to community health, Philadelphia, 1977, J.B. Lippincott Co.

Emery, F.E., editor: Systems thinking, Baltimore, 1969, Penguin Books, Inc.

Falk, L.A. Community participation in the neighborhood health center, Journal of the National Medical Association 61:493-497, November 1969.

Fienberg, S.E.: Perspective: Canada as a social report, Social Indicators Research 2:153-174, 1975.

Fienberg, S.E., and Goodman, L.A.: Social Indicators, 1973: statistical considerations. In Dusen, R.A., (ed.), Social Indicators, 1973: A review symposium, Washington, D.C., 1974, Center for Coordination of Research on Social Indicators, Social Science Research Council.

Firestone, J.M.: The development of social indicators from content analysis of social documents, Policy Sciences 3(2):249-263, 1972.

Freeman, R.: Community health nursing practice, Philadelphia, 1979, W.B. Saunders Co.

Fromer, M.J.: Community health care and the nursing process, St. Louis, 1979, The C.V. Mosby Co.

Gaupp, P.G.: Authority, influence, and control in consultation, Community Mental Health Journal 2:205-210, 1966.

Gause, D.C., and Weinberg, G.M.: On systems education, General Systems Yearbook 18:137-146, 1973.

Gebbie, K.M.: Consultation contracts: their development and evaluation, American Journal of Public Health 60:1916-1920, October 1970.

Gibb, J.R.: The role of the consultant, The Journal of Social Issues 15:1-4, 1959.

Glaser, B.G., and Strauss, A.L.: The discovery of grounded theory: strategies for qualitative research, Chicago, 1967, Aldine Publishing Co.

Glidewell, J.C.: The entry problem in consultation, The Journal of Social Issues 15:51-59, 1959.

Goodstein, L.: Consultation with human service systems, Reading, Mass., 1978, Addison-Wesley Publishing Co., Inc.

Gray, W., Duhl, F.J., and Rizzo, N.D., editors: General systems theory and psychiatry, Boston, 1969, Little, Brown & Co.

Green, E., and others: Health education planning: a diagnostic approach, Palo Alto, Calif., 1980, Mayfield Publishing Co.

Hall, J.E., and Weaver, B.R.: Distributive nursing practice: a systems approach to community health, Philadelphia, 1977, J.B. Lippincott Co.

Hanchett, E.: Community health assessment: a conceptual tool kit, New York, 1979, John Wiley & Sons, Inc.

Hargraves, W.A., Atkisson, C.C., and Sorensen, J.E.: Resource materials for community mental health program evaluation, DHEW Pub. No. [ADM] 77-328, Rockville, Md., 1977, National Institute of Mental Health.

Hoff, W.: Resolving the health manpower crisis: systems approach to utilizing personnel, American Journal of Public Health 61:2491-2504, December 1971.

Jain, V.: Structural analysis of general systems theory, Behavioral Science 26:51-62, January 1981.

Kahn, S.: How people get power, New York, 1970, McGraw-Hill Book Co.

Klir, G., editor: Trends in general systems theory, New York, 1972, John Wiley & Sons, Inc.

Koestler, A., and Smithies, J.R., editors: Beyond reductionism: new perspectives in the life sciences, New York, 1969, Macmillan, Inc.

Kramer, R., and Specht, H.: Reading in community organizational practice, Englewood Cliffs, N.J., 1967, Prentice-Hall, Inc.

Laszlo, C.A., Levine, M.D., and Milsum, J.H.: A general systems framework for social systems, Behavioral Science 19(2):79-92, 1974.

Laszlo, E., editor: The relevance of general systems theory, New York, 1972, George Braziller, Inc.

Laszlo, E.: The systems view of the world, New York, 1972, George Braziller, Inc., Laszlo, E., editor: The world system models, norms, variations, New York, 1973, George Braziller, Inc.

Laszlo, E.: The meaning and significance of general systems theory, Behavioral Science 20:9-22, January 1975.

Lippitt, G.L.: Consulting with a national organization: a case study, The Journal of Social Issues 15:20-27, 1959.

Lippitt, G.L.: A study of the consultation process, The Journal of Social Issues 15:43-50, 1959.

Lippitt, G., and Lippitt, R.: The consulting process in action, LaJolla, Calif., 1978, University Associates.

Lippitt, R.: Dimensions of the consultant's job, The Journal of Social Issues 15:5-12, 1959.

Lippitt, R., Watson, J., and Westley, B.: The dynamics of planned change, New York, 1958, Harcourt, Brace & World, Inc.

Luther, T., and Brewer, W.: Stimulating community action in health, Nursing Outlook 18:41, May 1970.

Maxwell, A.E.: Basic statistics in behavioral research, Baltimore, 1970, Penguin Books, Inc.

Merry, U., and Allerhand, M.E.: Developing teams and organizations: a practical handbook for managers and consultants, Reading, Mass., 1977, Addison-Wesley Publishing Co., Inc.

Michael, J.R., editor: Working the system: a comprehensive manual for citizen access to federal agencies, New York, 1977, Basic Books, Inc., Publishers.

Miller, J.: Living systems: basic concepts, Behavioral Science 10:193-237, July 1965.

Miller, J.: Living systems, New York, 1977, McGraw-Hill Book Co.

Morgerstern, O.: On the accuracy of economic observations, Princeton, N.J., 1963, Princeton University Press.

Moynihan, D.P.: Maximum feasible misunderstanding: community action in the war on poverty, New York, 1969, The Free Press.

Navarro, V.: A systems approach to health planning, Health Services Research 4:96-111, Summer 1969.

Office of Economic Opportunity: The comprehensive neighborhood health services program: guidelines, Health Services Office, Communty Action Program, Washington, D.C., 1968, Office of Economic Opportunity.

Parsons, T.: The social system, Glencoe, Ill., 1958, Free Press.

Parsons, T., and others: Theories of society, New York, 1961, The Free Press.

Parsons, T., and Shels, E.A.: Toward a general theory of action, Cambridge, Mass., 1951, Harvard University Press.

Perkins, M.: Community, establishment, and power, New York State Journal of Medicine 70:442-445, February 1, 1970.

Pertman, R., and Gurin, A.: Community organization and social planning, New York, 1972, John Wiley & Sons, Inc.

Pierce, L.M.: Usefulness of a systems approach for problem conceptualization and investigation, Nursing Research **21**:509-513, November-December 1972.

Powers, P.S., and Girgenti, J.R.: Analysis of a system, Journal of Psychiatric Nursing and Mental Health Services **16**:17-22, July 1978.

Rapoport, A.: Modern systems theory: an outlook for coping with change, General Systems Yearbook **15**:15-25, 1970.

Reinhardt, A.M., and Quinn, M.D.: Family-centered community nursing: a socio-cultural framework, vol. 1, St. Louis, 1973, The C.V. Mosby Co.

Reinhardt, A.M., and Quinn, M.D.: Family-centered community nursing: a sociocultural framework, vol. 2, St. Louis, 1980, The C.V. Mosby Co.

Robbins, P.R., Spencer, E.C., and Frank, D.A.: Some factors influencing the outcome of consultation, American Journal of Public Health **60**(3):524-534, March 1970.

Rosen, G.: Public health: then and now—the first neighborhood health center, its rise and fall, American Journal of Public Health **61**:1620-1637, 1971.

Ross, M.: Community organization: theory, principle, and practice, ed. 2, New York, 1967, Harper & Row, Publishers, Inc.

Ross, D.K.: A public citizen's action manual, New York, 1973, Grossman Publishers.

Schatzman, L., and Strauss, A.L.: Field research: strategies for a natural sociology, Englewood Cliffs, N.J., 1973, Prentice-Hall, Inc.

Schein, E.A.: Process consultation: its roles in organization development, Reading, Mass., 1969, Addison-Wesley Publishing Co., Inc.

Schindler-Rainman, E., and Lippitt, R.: Team training for community change: concepts, goals, strategies, and skills, Fairfax, Va., 1972, Learning Resources Corp.

Schulberg, H.E., Sheldon, A., and Baker, F., editors: Program evaluation in the health fields, New York, 1969, Behavioral Publications, Inc.

Sedgwick, R.: The role of the process consultant, Nursing Outlook **21**:773-775, 1973.

Shannon, C.E., and Weaver, W.: The mathematical theory of communication, Urbana, Ill., 1949, University of Illinois Press.

Shrode, W.A., and Voich, D.: Organization and management: basic systems concepts, Homewood, Ill., 1974, Richard D. Irwin, Inc.

Signell, K.A., and Scott, P.A.: Training in consultation: a crisis in role transition, Community Mental Health Journal **8**:149-160, May 1972.

Silverman, M., and Lee, P.R.: Pills, profits, and politics, Berkeley, Calif., 1974, University of California Press.

Silverman, W.H.: Some factors related to consultee satisfaction with consultation, American Journal of Community Psychology **2**(3):303-311, September 1974.

Steele, S.M: Contemporary approaches to program evaluation and their implications for evaluating programs for disadvantaged adults, Washington, D.C., 1977, Administrative Resources Division, Capitol Publications, Inc.

Stephenson, P.S.: Judging the effectiveness of a consultation program to a community agency, Community Mental Health Journal **9**:253-259, 1973.

Suchman, E.A.: Evaluative research: principles and practice in public service and social action programs, New York, 1967, Russell Sage Foundation.

Tageson, C.W., and Corazzini, J.G.: A collaborative model for consultation and paraprofessional development, Professional Psychology **5**:191-197, May 1974.

Tieman, G.: Toward collaborative mental health consultation, Journal of Religion and Health **9**:371-376, October 1970.

Vickers, G.: Freedom in a rocking boat, London, 1970, Penguin Books, Ltd.

Von Bertalanffy, L.: General systems theory foundations, development, and application, New York, 1968, George Braziller, Inc.

Von Bertalanffy, L.: Perspectives on general systems theory, New York, 1975, George Braziller, Inc.

Von Bertalanffy, L.: Robots, men, and minds, New York, 1967, George Braziller, Inc.

Von Gigch, J.P.: Applied general systems theory, New York, 1978, Harper & Row, Publishers, Inc.

Von Neumann, J.: Theory of self-reproducing automata, Urbana, Ill., 1966, University of Illinois Press.

Watkins, E.L., Holland, T.P., and Ritvo, R.A.: Evaluating the impact of program consultation in health services, Cleveland, Ohio, 1975, Human Services Design Laboratory, School of Applied Social Sciences, Case Western Reserve University.

Watzlawick, P., Weakland, J.N., and Fisch, R.: Change: principles of problem formation and problem resolution, New York, 1974, W.W. Norton & Co., Inc.

Weiner, N.: Human use of human beings: cybernetics, New York, 1967, Avon Books.

Weiner, N.: Cybernetics, New York, 1974, John Wiley & Sons, Inc.

Weiss, C.H.: Evaluation research: methods of assessing program effectiveness, Englewood Cliffs, N.J., 1972, Prentice-Hall, Inc.

Werley, H.H., and others, editors: Health research: the systems approach, New York, 1976, Springer Publishing Co., Inc.

Wolfe, H.E.: Consultation: role, function, and process, Mental Hygiene **50:**132-134, 1966.

Zald, M., editor: Organizing for community welfare, Chicago, 1967, Quadrangle/The New York Times Book Co.

Zusman, J., and Davidson, D.L., editors: Practial aspects of mental health consultation, Springfield, Ill., 1972, Charles C Thomas, Publisher.

INDEX